I QUIT SUGAR

with *Sarah Wilson*

SLOW COOKER COOKBOOK

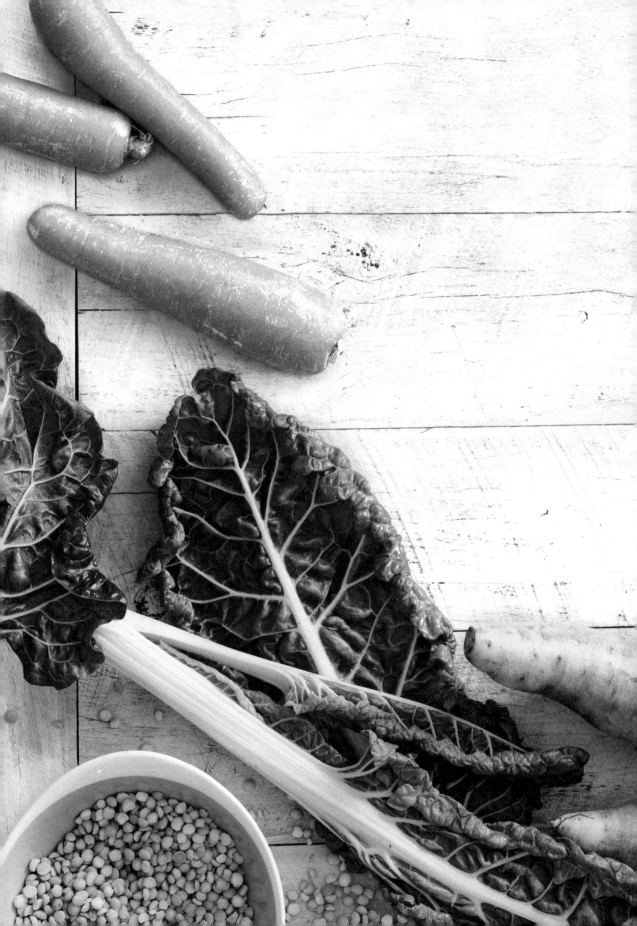

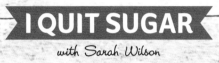

I QUIT SUGAR

with *Sarah Wilson*

SLOW COOKER COOKBOOK

**EASY, NUTRITIOUS
SLOW-COOKER RECIPES
FOR BUSY FOLK
& FAMILIES**

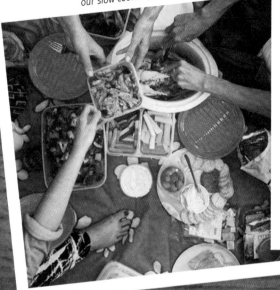

The team at the moonlight cinemas eating our slow-cooker creations.

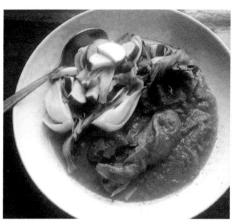

Vietnamese Chicken Curry was on the menu for lunch at the office.

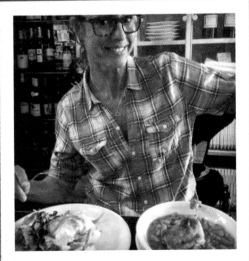

When I travel I seek out slow-cooked meals. Here I am in London eating duck cassoulet.

Some of my and the IQS Team's slow-cooker creations shared at I Quit Sugar HQ.

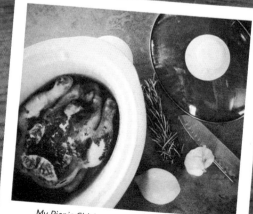

My Picnic Chicken with Lemony Gremolata (cooked on the bench at work!).

CONTENTS

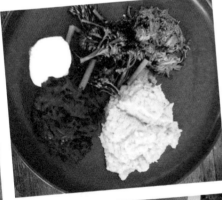

BBQ Pulled Pork with leftovers from the fridge.

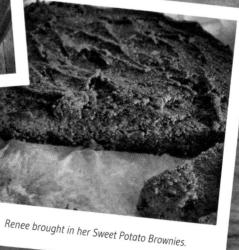

Renee brought in her Sweet Potato Brownies.

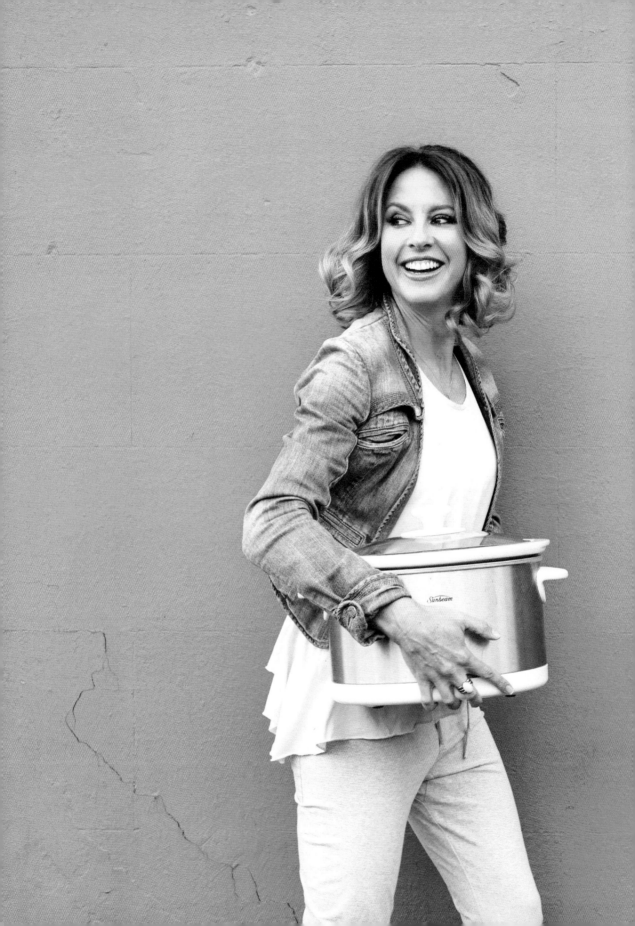

AN INTRODUCTORY CHAT

I quit sugar . . . and fell in love with my slow cooker.

When you quit sugar, as I did in 2011, a few interesting things happen. You get well. And you get clear. You stop snacking and a genuine, balanced appetite returns. Or as I like to say, you find 'food freedom'. It also means you stop eating crap.

When you quit sugar, you're essentially quitting processed foods.

Plus it gets you cooking, which I personally think is one of the most underrated benefits of this whole thing. As *New York Times* journalist Michael Pollan says, cooking is the best way to reclaim your health from big food.

'But cooking takes too much time. It's so much bother. And it's expensive,' comes the cry. Not so, my friends, if you have a slow cooker! I bought my first electric slow cooker for $39 around the same time I quit sugar, funnily enough. As I ventured into what was virgin territory back then (there were really no cookbooks or programmes available, nor websites sharing recipes) I found the easiest way to eat simply and sustainably was with this nifty kitchen device. Seriously, a slow cooker is sustainable in every sense (we explain how and why it saves time, money and the environment later on).

And it allows you to stop eating crap . . . for good.

At I Quit Sugar HQ, the team has badgered me for a Slow Cooker Cookbook for some time. We've gradually included slow-cooker recipes in our online 8-Week Programme and on IQuitSugar.com. But a stack of you seemed hungry for more. So I happily relented. For this cookbook, however, I got the IQS team to help me develop and test a number of the recipes. We bought a bunch of cookers and all set to IQS-ifying our nostalgic family meals, adjusting the recipes to fit my IQS principles.

Thus, I Quit Sugar slow-cooker recipes:

- **Contain no or very low sugar.** The desserts and 'sweet' recipes use fructose-free sweeteners (apart from whole fruits). But, as I like to remind everyone often: even these 'safe' sweeteners can continue sweet cravings and some science suggests glucose comes with its own health issues. So we keep all sweeteners to an absolute minimum.

- **Avoid other hidden sugars.** Many slow-cooker cookbooks rely on commercial sauces and plenty of canned tomatoes for flavour. Ours doesn't. We minimise the use of tomato purées and other tomato products and substitute with different clever options.

- **Are one-pot wonders.** Most of our recipes are designed to be thrown into the cooker in one hit, no extra steps or pans required.

- **Are designed for busy people.** They require 8–9 hours of cooking – whack it on in the morning and dinner is ready by the time you get home from work or school or a day tied up with kids. Better still, where possible, we show you how to prepare your meal the night before so that you only have to hit 'start' in the morning as you race out the door. Most of the meals are freezable, too, making them perfect for busy people.

- **Are designed to feed six.** All main meals will easily feed six and may leave you with some tasty leftovers for tomorrow's lunch or next week's stew.

- **Are great for singles.** Cook in bulk, divide into six portions and freeze for fast mid-week meals for one.

- **Prioritise dense nutrition.** We pack every meal with more than enough macro and micronutrients, using extra vegetables and the best quality proteins.

- **Are cheap-as.** There is a list of budget recipes for you on page 21.

- **Include a few extend-your-repertoire quirks.** I like to throw in a curve ball or two in all my cookbooks. This time I hope to get you all into the joy of cooking and eating offal. Trust me, we've made these recipes very appealing!

As a final little thought as I sit here with my Mum's Steak and Kidney Stew (see page 103) simmering away (I'm testing it on my family to get their feedback), I've realised that the true joy of slow cooking is in its *slow and low* approach. Enjoying food should be languid and mindful – not about blasting the daylights out of it. There's joy, too, in the communal experience it brings. All of which, I guess, continues the I Quit Sugar message, which is a gentle experiment that you share with those around you as you see fit. Right?

Happy slow cooking everyone!

Sarah (and the I Quit Sugar Team)

Sarah
xx

WHY USE A SLOW COOKER?

Where do we start? We're obsessed with our slow cookers! Here's why:

It's super economical: Slow cooking actually demands the use of cheap or secondary cuts of meat: neck, shins, cheeks and chuck. These cuts are often a third of the cost of the more 'fashionable' cuts. The low and slow method of cooking also requires less meat as it's often bulked out with veggies and the maximum amount of nutrients are extracted from the meat. Slow cookers are cheap to buy – about £20–40 in most department stores.

It's ethical: How so? We use cuts of the animal (again neck, shins etc) that are often not valued by other consumers and often go to waste.

It's energy efficient: A slow cooker uses about the same amount of electricity as a traditional light bulb and, so, if you are cooking a full meal, you'll use less electricity than your oven. Also, since you leave it on during the day, it's using power from the grid at a low-demand time.

It's convenient: Slow cooking has to be the most time-saving method of cooking out there. Simply dump all your ingredients in the cooker and go about your business for the day. No stirring, no checking, no fancy tricks. Just drop the ingredients in and go!

Did we mention that 80 per cent of the recipes in this book are one-pot wonders?!

For loads of easy and clever recipes check out the Weekday Dump 'n' Run chapter (see page 59).

It's tastier: Cooking secondary cuts of meat in a slow cooker can result in the most succulent, melt-in-the-mouth dish. The slow cooking of the protein allows the meat to gently fall away from the bone without drying up or shrinking, ergo, more juicy meat for everyone. The long, slow cooking extracts loads of flavour from the ingredients you are using.

It's all about dense nutrition and better digestive health: The slow-cooker cuts are often the most nutritious. These cuts are from muscles on the animal that contain the greatest amount of connective tissue, which, when slow cooked, dissolves into gelatin. Gelatin works wonders for repairing the gut and aids digestion in general.

> **DID YOU KNOW?**
>
> High temperatures and steam can account for the loss of as much as 30 per cent of the vitamin content of some vegetables. Using the slow cooker will allow you to preserve the vitamins and minerals in your food.

HOW TO BUY YOUR MEAT

The beauty of slow cooking is that it requires you to use cheap cuts of meat. You don't use sirloin in a slow cooker. You use the tougher and bonier cuts, the bits most folk don't buy. And, so, they're cheaper. Which – as I say often – means you can then make more ethical meat-buying decisions, like paying more for organic and pasture-fed.

Always buy from sustainable suppliers

Check the farming practices used by your suppliers, supermarkets or local farmers are sustainable. This means they consider wastage, water use, land degradation, transportation and their overall carbon footprint.

How to buy beef

Go for pasture-fed. Pasture-fed animals forage on grass and tend not to be treated with hormones or antibiotics.

> ### DID YOU KNOW?
> Animals under strain and stress when slaughtered produce tougher meat. Consider the practices of your suppliers and butchers when doing your shop.

Go for organic. Non-organic beef can be treated with growth-promoting hormones. It might say a lot to you that the European Union has banned growth hormones and deemed them a health risk.

We've highlighted the cuts of beef that we've used in this book. They're the most nutritious and economical for you.

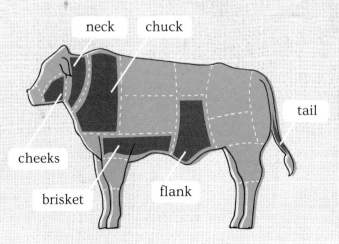

Beef/ox liver: Offal is incredibly dense in nutrition, loaded with protein, vitamins A and D, iron and folic acid. It's also dirt-cheap and one of the most underrated parts of the animal. For more info and recipes on offal, check out the offal section (see page 99).

Brisket: Cut from the breast or lower chest of beef or veal. Brisket is ideal for slow cooking as all the connective tissues break down and tenderise over time. If you're new to brisket try the Beef Brisket 'n' Beer with Gravy (see page 88), you can't go wrong.

Chuck steak/roast: This is a thick cut of meat from the shoulder of the cow. It's an inexpensive cut with a rich flavour. Use it as stewing meat as I do in my mum's Hungarian Goulash (see page 49).

Beef cheeks: Found in the facial cheek of a cow – not the bum! They're tough and contain plenty of connective tissues, but when they're slow cooked they taste incredible. I'd recommend the slow-cooked Chinese Beef Cheeks (see page 108) if you're new to cooking cheeks.

WHY GRAIN-FED BEEF AIN'T GREAT

Grain-fed beef can present a host of ethical, health and environmental issues (the animals are kept in small lots, the grains increase the omega-6 count of the meat, and using fertile land for animal grain is wasteful). Having said that, in Australia, unlike most of the world, most lamb and 70 per cent of beef is pasture-fed and raised on arid rangelands where nothing else can be grown (no fertile land is wasted). Hoorah!

The UK is much the same with most beef and lamb being grass-fed and occasionally grain-finished.

However, in the US and the EU most beef is grain-fed and there are conflicting issues with suppliers labelling meat 'grass-fed' when it isn't.

DID YOU KNOW?

Some restaurants actually sell their steak as 'grain-fed' (with wheat, soy, corn). Why? Grain-fed beef, such as Wagyu or Kobe, is said to produce fatty, marbled meat, which is considered fashionable in high-end restaurants because of its distinctive flavour and texture. Don't be sold by this!

How to buy lamb

Go for pasture-fed. In Australia and the UK, most lamb is pasture-fed.

Go for organic. Where possible buy organic lamb to avoid growth-promoting hormones and nitrates, used during the processing of meat, contaminating your food.

We've highlighted the cuts of lamb that we've used in this book. They're the most nutritious and economical for you.

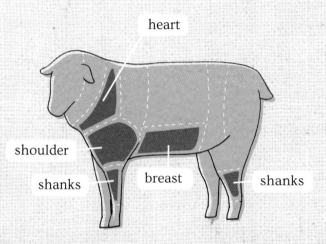

Shanks: A shank is the portion around the leg bone beneath the knee. Lamb shanks are commonly used in slow cooking as the meat breaks down and tenderises over time. Shanks can be rather large, often 400 grams each. I like to buy one or two, cook them up, shred the meat and separate into 3–4 portions for meals later on. New to cooking lamb shanks? Try the Lemon and Cinnamon Lamb Shanks with Lemony Gremolata (see page 67).

Lamb shoulder: Lamb shoulder is inexpensive and can be bought with the bone intact or removed. We recommend you buy it intact where possible in order to extract maximum flavour and meat. However, if your slow cooker is quite small it's best to go for a cut with the bone removed. A whole shoulder will easily serve six people and a half shoulder will serve 3–4 people. Cook slowly until the meat falls away from the bone. I recommend you try the Spiced Lamb Shoulder (see page 54).

Lamb heart and sweetbreads: See the advice on lamb hearts and sweetbreads in the offal section (see page 99).

How to buy pork

Pork is loaded with nutritional benefits including protecting the liver, detoxifying the lungs and even cleansing the system of cholesterol. To read up on its connection to longevity visit SarahWilson.com.

Go for free-range (outdoor-reared). This is generally the most ethically raised type of pork as the animals have the greatest amount of space and time to roam freely before slaughter.

Go for organic. This will ensure no recycled food waste (that could risk bacterial contamination) is permitted in the feed system, guaranteeing you're eating the healthiest and safest pork available.

DID YOU KNOW?

There is no legal definition for free-range pork in Australia, the US, the UK, the EU or Asia so your best option is to speak directly to the supplier or your butcher and find out more information on where your meat is coming from.

We've highlighted the cuts of pork that we've used in this book. They're the most nutritious and economical for you.

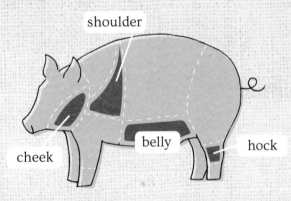

Ham hock: A ham hock, also known as the pork knuckle, is the joint between the leg and the foot. Ham hock keeps on giving and can be used a few times over for flavour in stews and soups. Try adding it to a comfort classic like Classic Pea and Ham Soup (see page 45).

Pork belly: This is a very fatty piece of meat often used in Asian cooking with plentiful amounts of sugary seasonings. Check out our 'Maple Syrup' Pork Belly with Pecans (see page 122) for an easy and clever twist on a classic Asian favourite, sans sugar.

Pork shoulder: This is a common cut of meat for pulled pork but it's often overlooked by customers as it needs around eight hours cooking time to achieve a shredded texture. For your own delicious pulled pork experience try the 'Barbecued' Pulled Pork with Cauliflower Cream (see page 111).

How to buy chicken

Go for organic. Many authorities say it's worth investing in organic poultry products over free-range. I tend to agree. I cook the whole chicken, often slowly, to extract as much nutrition as possible. I certainly don't want to be leaching residual chemicals into my soup too! To read up on why I believe organic chicken is the best choice for you and your family visit SarahWilson.com.

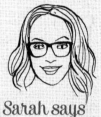

Sarah says

" Invest extra cash in organic chicken but make it affordable by buying cheaper cuts (not the breast!), or, better still, cooking the whole bird. You can even stretch things out by cooking up the bones after. See the recipe for Chicken Stock on page 28. "

THE DEAL WITH FREE-RANGE

The term 'free-range' is loosely regulated. 'Free-range' can legally be attached to an egg from a 10,000 chickens per hectare farm (0.25 square metre per bird). The best thing to do is research your supplier and find out what the conditions on the farm are like. Many farmers now have live cameras that allow you to see the conditions on the farm.

We've highlighted the cuts of chicken that we've used in this book. They're the most nutritious and economical for you.

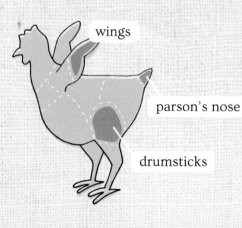

wings

parson's nose

drumsticks

Chicken wings: Wings are totally underrated. They're super cheap (even organic ones!), loaded with flavour and the bones and cartilage are soft enough to eat. These parts are where the minerals – particularly calcium, magnesium and potassium – are contained that feed, repair and calm the mucous lining in the small intestines and calm the nervous system.

Chicken drumsticks: Like chicken wings, drumsticks are considered less glamorous than the breast. But they're significantly cheaper in price and when cooked on the bone they're loaded with flavour and moisture. Dark meat is also better for you than the white as it contains more minerals than the breast.

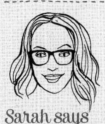

"I always eat the chicken skin. It contains the right fat-soluble vitamins and fatty acids to help my body properly metabolise the chicken meat."

Sarah says

Leftover chicken bones: For a cheap way to add in some dense nutrition ask your butcher for leftover bones and make your own stocks and broths. Often you can get bones for free or buy them for next to nothing. Chicken bones are loaded with gelatin, which is essential for digestion and repairing the gut.

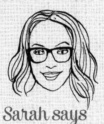

"I'll often scrape all the leftover chicken bones off everyone's plates and pour them straight into a stock pot or slow cooker as the base of my Chicken Stock. Don't be afraid of this . . . you then boil them to bits!"

Sarah says

The deal with kangaroo meat

In Australia, roo meat has now become as commonplace in supermarkets as chicken or beef. Due to the increase in kangaroo numbers in Australia it has become necessary to commercially harvest 10–15 per cent of the population yearly to prevent economic and environmental damage. Rest assured, strict controls ensure that no more than the quota number is actually harvested.

Why eat it?

Kangaroo meat is super lean, rich in high-quality protein, a good source of zinc and an excellent source of iron (and cheap too!). It also contains conjugated linoleic acid (CLA); a fat which research shows has antioxidant properties and may help reduce body fat in humans. Save cash and enjoy some richly nutritious protein with the recipe for Roo Rogan Josh with a Cucumber Raita (see page 116).

WHAT ABOUT FISH?!

You won't find any fish recipes in this cookbook. IQS headquarters did some research, tested a few recipes and realised that fish and slow cooking don't really go together. We want this book to be loaded with punchy flavours and melt-in-your-mouth protein. We think you can achieve this easily and (quickly!) by pan-frying, poaching or oven-baking fish. If you're still fanging for some fish you can find some of our favourite recipes at IQuitSugar.com.

IT'S OFFAL GOOD
FOR YOU!

We've included a few recipes that use offal, or organs. Why?! Because they're densely nutritious, dirt cheap, flavoursome and sustainable. Before you start, a little lesson on the different types you'll be cooking with:

Liver

Liver is an excellent source of high-quality protein loaded with vitamin A and several B vitamins. It's also an excellent source of folic acid and iron as well as the number-one food source of copper.

Go for: Beef/ox, lamb, chicken or duck livers. Choose liver with no patches of grey colour and an inoffensive odour.

How to prepare: Chicken livers don't need soaking – simply rinse them under cold water for a couple of minutes and pat dry. Using a sharp knife, remove any exposed veins, ducts or connective tissue then use your fingers to peel away the outer membrane.

Kidney

Beef/ox kidneys are one of the most commonly used forms of offal. You can buy them quite cheaply from any good butcher. Eating a single portion is the equivalent to eating six large eggs or five bags of baby spinach.

Go for: Beef or lamb kidneys that are plump, deep red in colour and don't have a strong odour.

How to prepare: You can usually buy them pre-trimmed or ask your local butcher to do it for you. If you're preparing it yourself, use a sharp knife and cut the fat off the kidney. Soak in water and refrigerate for two hours prior to cooking to remove the odour. Slice it in half and cut around the membrane. Now you can trim the soft meat for your recipe. Discard the membrane and keep the fat to render down later and add to a stew. For some clever ways to use leftover fat see page 17.

Heart

Heart is a fairly muscly organ and can be likened to a cheaper version of steak or minced beef. Heart is super high in protein and a great source of thiamine, folate, selenium, phosphorus, zinc and several of the B vitamins.

Go for: Heart that is deep reddish brown with a thin layer of fat near the top. Where possible, choose heart that has come from grass-fed animals for better taste and nutritional benefits.

How to prepare: Ask your local butcher to trim the heart, as it can be tricky to do yourself. Heart is fairly delicate during the cooking process so cook it slowly. Try the Stuffed Lambs' Hearts (see page 105), a recipe from our General Manager, Zoe, for an IQS take on a classic.

Sweetbreads

Not to be confused with sweet bread, these are definitely offal. There are two types of sweetbreads, stomach sweetbreads (also known as heart or belly sweetbreads) from an animal's pancreas and neck sweetbreads from an animal's thymus gland.

Go for: Those that are white, fleshy and firm to the touch.

How to prepare: Sweetbreads should be soaked in several changes of cold water (refrigerated) for about an hour and a half to rid them of impurities – if you want them to be a creamy white colour, add a squeeze of lemon juice with each change of water. I experimented with sweetbreads for this book. You can try my recipe for Sweetbread Burritos on page 106.

GETTING STARTED

Buying an electric slow cooker

All the recipes in this book use an electric slow cooker. We promise you it's a small investment that will reward you tenfold. Most department stores sell a basic slow cooker for around £30.

When choosing a slow cooker go for:

- **An electric model.**
- **One with a 4.5 litre capacity** or as close to this size as possible. Every recipe in this book is made for this size slow cooker, however most recipes (except those from the Cakes and Puds chapter) will work in all sizes.
- **One with a timer** (optional). An automated timer allows for you to leave a slow cooker on all day or just a few hours and not have to return to switch it off. Not mandatory, but definitely handy.
- **One with a pre-browning feature** (optional). This will save you time cleaning pots and pans and can enhance the flavour of the final product. That said, none of the IQS team use one and our recipes don't require pre-browning.

My slow cooker is bigger/smaller than 4.5 litres

If your slow cooker is slightly bigger or smaller than 4.5 litres, that's fine – just adjust the recipe to suit by adding more or less of the core ingredients. You may need to increase the quantities in the cakes, tarts and batter recipes if you have a bigger slow cooker to ensure they don't burn.

> **TRICKY TIP**
>
> Slow cookers work best when filled to two-thirds of capacity.

I don't have a slow cooker (or how to slow cook in an oven)

You can still enjoy all of the recipes in this book without an electric slow cooker, with a bit of tweaking here and there.

What to cook in: We recommend a casserole dish – a double-handled, deep ovenproof dish that has a tight-fitting lid made from cast iron, glass, ceramic or any other heatproof and flameproof material.

How to slow cook using an oven: Simply seal the meat in a deep casserole dish on the stovetop until lightly browned, chuck in the additional ingredients and place the pot, with the lid on, in the oven for the adjusted cooking time.

For an easy cooking conversion guide see our table:

SLOW COOKER	CONVENTIONAL OVEN 160°C/GAS 3
1–1 ½ hours on high 4–5 hours on low	30–60 minutes
3–4 hours on high 6–8 hours on low	1–2 hours
4–6 hours on high 10–12 hours on low	3–4 hours

The low setting on a slow cooker is between 79–80°C/176°F and the high setting on a slow cooker is between 90–93°C/199°F. If you want to use the oven like you would a slow cooker you can set it to these temperatures and cook to the recommended time on the recipe.

SLOW COOKERS VS PRESSURE COOKERS

Both slow cookers and pressure cookers have their pros and cons from a convenience point of view but when it comes to nutritional benefits we think slow cooking is the way to go. A slow cooker maintains the integrity of the food whereas pressure cooking does just that – puts pressure on the food. Cooking food under extreme heat renders the protein and veggies void of many essential nutrients and obliterates the enzymes needed to help your gut digest food. Our take? Go low and slow.

NINE IMPORTANT THINGS TO KNOW

1. **Less is more:** Don't add as much water as conventionally cooked recipes indicate. When you're using a slow cooker the liquid doesn't reduce in the same way that it would on a stovetop. Generally 1 cup (250 ml) of liquid is enough for most recipes unless it contains a starch like rice or pasta.

2. **Lid on is best:** Always cook the meal with the lid on, except in the case of baking, or cooking puddings where you may need to remove the lid for a period of time.

3. **Keep your mitts off:** Your slow cooker works best when undisturbed. You'll need to add an additional 20 minutes on high each time you lift the lid. If you need to stir, do it in the last few hours.

4. **Don't stress about cooking times:** The times in this book are approximate. Timing is not critical to a dish's success, however the longer a meal cooks the better the flavour and the more tender the meat will be.

5. **Some peace of mind:** Even if you leave your slow cooker on for 12 hours the meat won't burn, stick or dry up.

6. **Some foods don't belong in a slow cooker:** Avoid slow cooking crisp green veggies, noodles, Chinese vegetables and pasta. These ingredients are best served on the side. Check out the A Few Clever Sides chapter (see page 123) for some tasty options.

7. **Order matters:** It's generally best to put veggies in first with meat on top unless specified.

8. **Frozen veggies:** Can be tossed straight in. No need to defrost.

9. **The Golden Rule:** Most casseroles with meat and vegetables need about 8 hours on low.

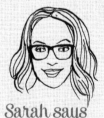

Sarah says

"There's no need to pre-brown. A lot of slow cooker recipes suggest browning meat in a separate pan before placing in the slow cooker, in part to render the fat, allowing some of it to drain away. In most cases, I reckon it's a waste of time and pans. In the few cases where browning makes sense I tend to ensure we use the browning pan again later to make gravy etc."

HOW TO USE LEFTOVERS

If there's one thing you need to take away from this cookbook it's the beauty of leftovers. Every recipe will produce more than enough food to feed you and your friends or family. Plus more!

Here, we've listed some ways to store and use up leftovers. We've also added a '3 Ways' stamp for those recipes that can be turned into two more equally satisfying dishes.

1) How to freeze cooked leftover portions

- We like to use plastic ziplock bags for freezing individual portions. BPA-free plastic containers are also a good option. The good news: plastic ziplock bags are now safer (no longer made from PVC).

- If you've made a large batch of soup, stew or curry for the week, dish each portion into freezer-friendly, microwave-safe containers. Remove from the freezer in the morning and defrost in the fridge throughout the day.

- Defrost foods in the fridge, not on the bench. The slower you defrost the closer it resembles its pre-frozen state.

- If you have leftover meat, shred and freeze in 1-cup portions (or 150 g of meat per person) in ziplock bags or freezer-friendly containers. If you're likely to microwave leftover portions make sure the container is microwave safe too.

- When defrosting and cooking leftovers, remove from the freezer, defrost in the fridge and add into the slow cooker towards the end of the cooking process to keep meat moist.

- If you want to jazz up your leftovers try some ideas from the Pimp My Stew section on page 19.

- Always label and date your containers to make it easier for yourself later on.

How long will my cooked leftovers last in the fridge or freezer?

		FRIDGE	FREEZER
Soups and stews	Vegetable	5 days	3–4 months
	Meat	3–4 days	2 months
Leftovers	Meat or poultry	3–4 days	2 months
	Vegetable-based	5 days	3 months
Pâté and offal		1–2 days	2 months
Cakes and slices		2–4 days	3 months

2) How to freeze and use leftover staples

- Freeze cooked or raw bones in large ziplock bags. This means next time you make stock you can remove them from the freezer and place straight into the slow cooker with all the other stock ingredients.

- Freeze leftover purées, stock and sauces. Measure them out in ½-cup (125 ml) portions, ready to use in your next slow cooker meal.

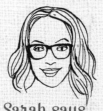

Sarah says

" I pour leftover wine or stock into my ice-lolly moulds. They're exactly a ½ cup (125 ml) capacity, making it easy for me to store and use. "

- Par-cook leftover veggies that look like they're wilting. Freeze them in freezer-friendly containers or ziplock bags, ensuring all air is removed. Toss veggies straight from the freezer into a slow cooker soup or stew to bulk it out.

- Freeze fresh herbs in ice-cube trays with leftover oil/fat, stock or wine. Pop out a few cubes and place straight into a slow-cooked soup or stew when you're after some extra flavour.

- Spoon leftover tomato purée or curry paste into ice-cube trays. Freezing stops them growing mould in the fridge. Use in slow cooker meals down the track.

- Once you have frozen leftovers in ice-cube trays pop them out into another container or ziplock bag to free up your tray again.

TRICKY TIP

A full freezer is an economical one. Why? Because solids freeze at a lower temperature than air, requiring less electricity to keep the freezer cold.

- Don't throw out excess liquid. If your stew is too runny ladle excess liquid out of the slow cooker and freeze in ½-cup (125 ml) portions or store in the fridge for up to a week in a glass jar. Use instead of stock (watered down a little) in soups and stews or drink as a broth.

- Got leftover mince? Make a batch of meat into meatballs or patties and freeze uncooked, placing greaseproof paper between each patty.

- Freeze your nuts. To avoid your nuts and seeds going rancid place them in ziplock bags ensuring excess air is removed. Freeze for up to six months.

3) How to use leftover fat

We don't have a problem with fat – you can read up on our thoughts on IQuitSugar.com. Good saturated fats have a multitude of health benefits and give food flavour, but a few of the recipes in this book will produce excess fat and oil. This is simply the nature of slow cooking – the gelatinous residue isn't rendered away like it is in oven baking or pan-frying.

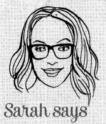

Sarah says

" With very fatty cuts of meat like pork belly, before serving up a dish I remove the lid and skim the fat off the surface. You can even cool it down completely to remove the excess fat – this makes the process easier as the fat will solidify at cooler temperatures. "

- Freeze leftover fat in a glass jar or ice-cube tray for up to one year. Whenever you need it pop out a cube and use it to sauté vegetables instead of oil or butter. Some people like to render their fat from scratch.
- Make popcorn and drizzle with the excess fat.
- Spread on the outside part of a grilled cheese sandwich instead of butter for a golden crunch.
- If you're game, try making your own soap. There are plenty of video tutorials online to help you with this.

A WORD ON FAT

As you flick through the recipes you'll notice there is very little additional oil or fat. This is because slow cooking allows fat to slowly fall away from the protein resulting in an incredibly rich residue in the sauce or base of your slow cooker. With some dishes we encourage you to 'skim off the fat' or 'pan-fry your meat' beforehand to avoid the overly fatty remains sitting on the surface of your meal.

STORE CUPBOARD ESSENTIALS

A handy guide of all the essentials you'll need in your larder, fridge and freezer to enjoy the recipes in this book.

- ❏ Beef, pork, lamb, chicken and offal. You can read up on the best cuts to buy on page 4.
- ❏ Sweet potato OR pumpkin
- ❏ Organic stock. You can make your own chicken, beef and vegetable stock using the recipes in the Stupidly Simple Staples chapter.
- ❏ Tomato purée
- ❏ Canned tomatoes (whole or chopped)
- ❏ Organic dried legumes OR canned legumes
- ❏ Coconut milk OR coconut cream
- ❏ Fresh flat-leaf parsley and coriander
- ❏ Tamari OR soy sauce
- ❏ White wine
- ❏ Apple cider vinegar
- ❏ Granulated stevia
- ❏ Rice malt syrup
- ❏ Arrowroot OR cornflour OR plain flour (gluten-free or otherwise)
- ❏ Dried herbs and spices (we picked a few key ones that form the basis of many of the recipes throughout this book).

  - ❏ Smoked sweet paprika or regular paprika
  - ❏ Peppercorns or cloves
  - ❏ Bay leaves
  - ❏ Thyme
  - ❏ Ground allspice
  - ❏ Cayenne pepper
  - ❏ Curry powder
  - ❏ Ground nutmeg
  - ❏ Ground ginger
  - ❏ Dried mixed herbs
  - ❏ Ground turmeric
  - ❏ Ground coriander
  - ❏ Dried chilli flakes or ground chilli powder
  - ❏ Sea salt
  - ❏ Freshly ground black pepper
  - ❏ Cinnamon

A NOTE ON TOMATOES

Yes, tomatoes contain sugar – about ¾ teaspoon per medium tomato. Traditionally, slow cooker recipes rely a lot on canned tomatoes and purée, sometimes up to two cans (8–10 tomatoes). We use them a little, but work to no more than ½ tomato per serve, with no more than ½ teaspoon of tomato purée per serve.

PIMP MY STEW

We've come up with some ideas to help you jazz up the leftovers from your slow cooker stews and curries.

	HERE'S WHAT TO DO
Turn it into a pie.	Spoon the stew mixture into an ovenproof pie dish. Cover with puff pastry and use a fork to press down the edges of the pastry around the dish. Prick pastry with a fork 3–4 times and glaze with egg wash (one egg whisked). Bake in the oven at 200°C/gas 6 for 25–30 minutes or until the pastry is puffed and golden.
Add dumplings.	The dumplings on page 104 can easily be added to any stew or casserole for a contrasting texture and to help mop up all those yummy juices.
Create a san choi bow wrap.	Pull apart an iceberg lettuce. Fill each lettuce cup with the leftover mince or stew mixture (you may need to drain away some of the sauce). To eat, wrap the lettuce leaves up into a parcel. Serve with any leftover Cucumber Raita (see page 116) or a homemade Asian dipping sauce of soy/tamari, chilli, ginger, lime and rice malt syrup.
Do a 'cheat's' stew and mash.	Throw some sweet potato or pumpkin into the slow cooker with the stew. Cover and cook until the veggies are cooked through and have collapsed, then serve. Alternatively, try the Shanky Shepherd's Pie (see page 68) approach.
Turn it into a lasagne.	Layer excess stew between sheets of fresh lasagne or thin slices of aubergine and courgette. Top with cheese or a bechamel sauce. Cook in the oven on 180°C/gas 4 for 40 minutes or until the veggies or pasta are cooked through. (Note: you may need to cover with foil if the cheese is cooking faster than the veggies.) Serve with steamed greens.
Make a ragout.	Toss your warm leftover stew through cooked pasta and top with fresh herbs and parmesan shavings.
Have it for brekkie.	Crack a few eggs into your Sweet Pumpkin Sunday Beans (see page 39) and continue cooking on high in the slow cooker. Alternatively, fry some eggs and serve on top of the leftover meat from your stew. Serve with a side of wilted spinach.
Add some crunch.	If you're after a crunchy topping remove the pot from the slow cooker, top with breadcrumbs or grated cheese and place under the grill or in the oven until golden. (Make sure your slow-cooker pot is oven-safe!)

TROUBLESHOOTING QUESTIONS

A few quick fixes to some common slow-cooker queries:

If your stew, gravy or casserole looks dry: Remove the lid and pour in ½ cup (125 ml) of the base liquid (stock or water). Stir a little. Replace the lid and continue cooking for 20 minutes on high, then back to low.

If your stew, gravy or casserole is too thin: Combine a thickener (4 teaspoons cornflour, 2 teaspoons chia seeds or 4 teaspoons arrowroot flour) with 3 tablespoons cold water to form a paste. Remove the slow-cooker lid and stir through the paste. Cook dish with lid off for 30 minutes on high then turn the slow cooker back to low and continue cooking.

If there is too much liquid: Remove the lid and scoop out some of the liquid with a ladle. Don't throw this excess sauce away! Try some of the tips listed on page 16.

If your meat is dry: Unfortunately there isn't much you can do when this happens. Chances are the dish was cooked over the recommended time or you had your slow cooker on high for too long. Try shredding it up and using the meat in tacos or sandwiches with some homemade tzatziki or sugar-free sauce. We love shredded chicken in the Mexican Chilli Chicken Tacos (see page 77).

If the dish is too salty: The best thing you can do in this scenario is add more of the other ingredients to the dish and build up the flavours to cover up the salt.

If the flavour is too intense: Remove the meat from the dish and stir in 1 cup (250 ml) of stock. Cook the sauce for 30 minutes on high with the lid off. Return the meat, cover and continue cooking on low.

DID YOU KNOW?

Whenever you lift the lid off the slow cooker, the dish will drop in temperature. This means the dish will need to cook for longer – at least 20 minutes on high – in order to bring the dish back to the right temperature.

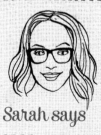

“ Rather than use flour, I use chia seeds or chia flakes to thicken a runny sauce . . . extra protein and nutrition!”

Sarah says

A LIST OF BUDGET MEALS

Here's a bunch of great, fuss-free recipes that won't break the bank!

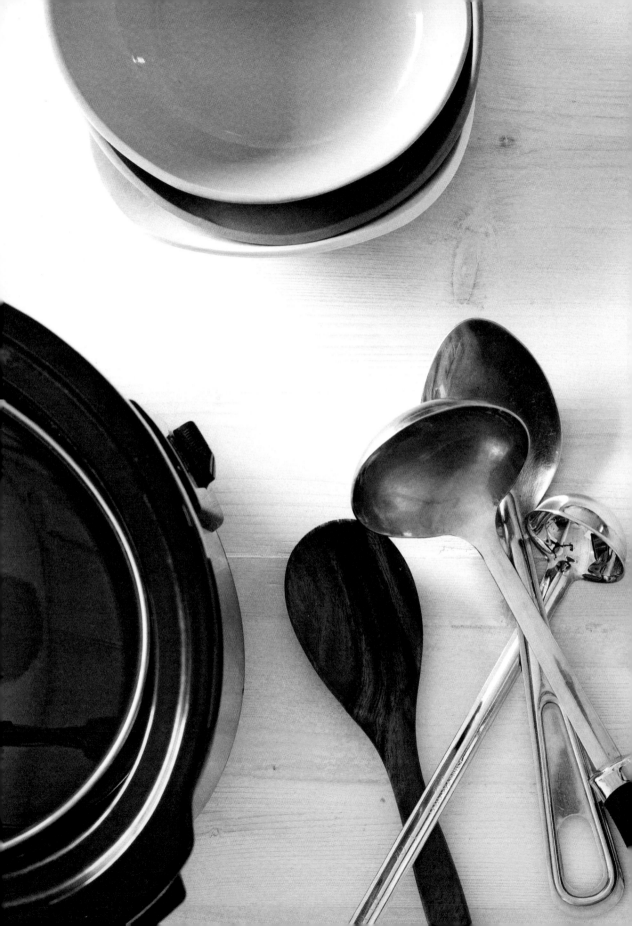

RECIPES

NAVIGATING THE RECIPES

We're almost there!

Just a few handy instructions on how to navigate the recipes in this book and then you'll be ready to cook.

These icons will point you in the right direction for recipes that suit your dietary needs.

P **Paleo:** Recipes that are grain and legume free. Note: our take on Paleo includes nuts and dairy.

GF **Gluten-free:** Recipes that don't contain gluten.

Veg **Vegetarian:** Meat-free recipes. Many of the recipes that do contain meat can be substituted with beans or other vegetarian proteins.

MF **Minimal Fructose:** Recipes with no stevia or rice malt syrup and a negligible amount of fructose will be marked with the minimal-fructose icon. These meals can be eaten while undertaking the 8-Week Programme.

 Freeze: Recipes that you can make a big batch of and keep for later. You'll see lots of these throughout the cookbook.

STUPIDLY SIMPLE STAPLES

A chapter brimful of the basic slow-cooker recipes you need to have in your repertoire.

BEGINNER'S
BEEF STOCK

This fail-safe beef stock can easily be made into a nourishing beef broth to drink daily.

MAKES 1.5 litres

PREPARATION TIME
5 minutes

COOKING TIME
10 hours on low
5 hours on high

1–2 kg soup bones, such as beef marrow and chopped beef shin (ask your butcher to chop them up for you)

2 stalks celery or celery leaves, roughly chopped

½ turnip, roughly chopped

1 carrot, roughly chopped

1 parsnip, roughly chopped

1 small onion, roughly chopped (don't bother peeling)

4 black peppercorns

cold water (approximately 6 cups/1.5 litres)

sea salt and freshly ground black pepper, to taste

IN THE MORNING

1. Remove any meat from the bones and chop finely. Place the bones in the slow-cooker insert with excess meat, vegetables and seasonings.

2. Fill the slow cooker two-thirds of the way to the top with cold water (don't fill to the top). Cover and cook overnight for 10 hours on low or 5 hours on high.

IN THE EVENING

1. Remove the bones from the slow cooker and strain the stock into a large pot or bowl.

2. When completely cool, skim the excess fat off the surface. (For ways to use leftover fats see page 17). Store the stock in the fridge in a sealed container for up to seven days or freeze in ½-cup (125 ml) portions.

TRICKY TIP

To make this a nourishing bone broth, as opposed to a stock, only cook the mixture for 6 hours on low before straining. Allow to cool. Store in 1-cup (250 ml) portions. Drink a cup daily for better digestion and gut health.

LEFTOVERS VEGETABLE STOCK

GF MF ❄ P Veg

MAKES
2 litres

PREPARATION TIME
5 minutes

COOKING TIME
8 hours on low
4 hours on high

4 cups (about 600 g) vegetable scraps (such as celery ends and leaves, onion trimmings, carrot tops)

2 litres water

sea salt and freshly ground black pepper, to taste

fresh herbs (optional)

IN THE MORNING

1. Place all the ingredients into the slow-cooker insert.

2. Cover and cook for 8 hours on low or 4 hours on high.

IN THE EVENING

1. Strain the stock, discard the veggie scraps and and allow to cool. Store in ½-cup (125 ml) portions in the freezer.

TOMATO SAUCE

GF ❄ P Veg

MAKES 3–4 cups
(0.7–1 litre)

PREPARATION TIME
5 minutes

COOKING TIME
5½ hours on low
3 hours on high

2 x 400 g cans diced tomatoes

½ onion, finely chopped

⅓ cup (75 ml) apple cider vinegar

1 tablespoon rice malt syrup

1 teaspoon ground allspice

1 teaspoon ground cinnamon

1 teaspoon ground cloves

1 teaspoon cayenne pepper

½ teaspoon sea salt

1. Combine all the ingredients in the slow-cooker insert.

2. Cover and cook for 5 hours on low or 2½ hours on high. Remove the mixture from the slow cooker and purée using a stick blender.

3. Return the puréed sauce to the slow-cooker insert and cook on high with the lid off for a further 30 minutes to thicken. Transfer the mixture to a clean glass jar and refrigerate for up to one month or freeze for up to three months.

CHICKEN STOCK

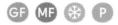

MAKES 3 litres

PREPARATION TIME
5 minutes

COOKING TIME
10 hours on low
5 hours on high

1 whole organic chicken (if you're friendly with your butcher, ask for some extra bony chicken bits; necks and feet as well) OR the leftover carcass of a whole organic chicken from a previous meal

splash of apple cider vinegar (or any vinegar)

2 carrots, roughly chopped

1 onion, roughly chopped (don't bother peeling)

2 stalks celery, roughly chopped

1 teaspoon black peppercorns

3 bay leaves

a few thyme sprigs (optional)

3–4 litres water (to cover chicken once in the slow cooker)

IN THE MORNING

1. Place all the ingredients in the slow-cooker insert. The water should cover the lot.

2. Cover and cook for 10 hours on low or 5 hours on high.

IN THE EVENING

1. Remove the chicken from the slow cooker. Strain the stock and allow to cool. Store in ½-cup (125 ml) portions in the freezer.

2. Shred the meat from the chicken carcass – it will pull away super easily from the bones. Portion out the meat into 5–6 serves in ziplock bags and stick in the freezer for sandwiches, salads and snacks. We use ours in the Mexican Chilli Chicken Tacos (see page 77).

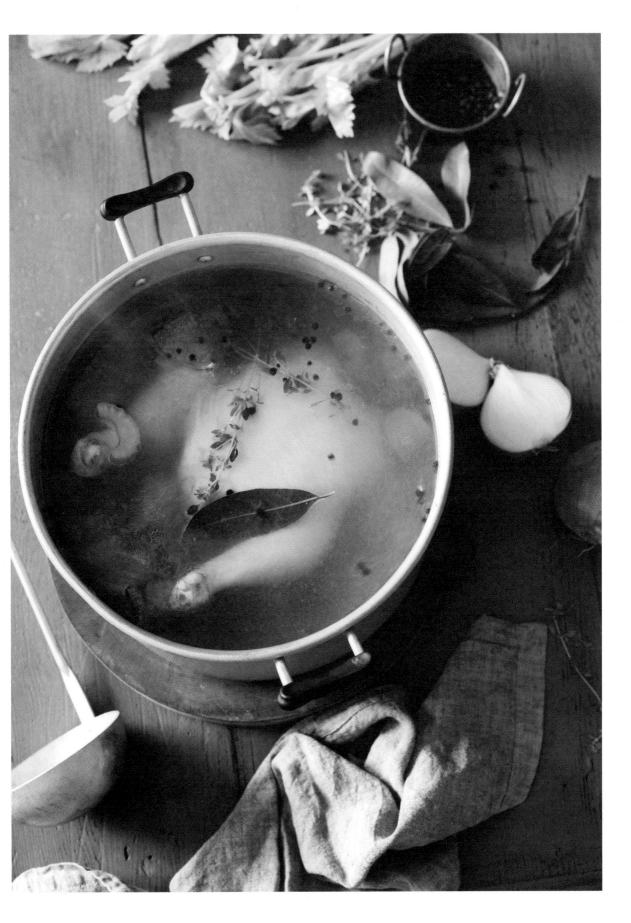

GLUTEN-FREE DAMPER

The success of this recipe may depend on the type of gluten-free flour you use; you may need to add more or less liquid than specified. If you want to achieve a golden crust, glaze the cooked damper with butter and cook in the oven at 180°C/gas 4 for 5–10 minutes.

SERVES 8

PREPARATION TIME
15 minutes

COOKING TIME
5–6 hours on low
3 hours on high

oil or butter, for greasing

4 cups (500 g) gluten-free self-raising flour

1 teaspoon sea salt

80 g butter, diced

1 teaspoon dried thyme

1 teaspoon dried rosemary

1 cup (250 ml) full-fat milk

½ cup (125 ml) water, if needed

1 teaspoon sesame seeds

1. Grease the inside of the slow-cooker insert and line with baking paper so that it reaches halfway up the sides.

2. Sift the flour and salt into a large bowl and rub in the butter with your fingertips until the mixture resembles breadcrumbs. Mix through the dried herbs.

3. Make a well in the centre of the flour mixture and pour in the milk.

4. Mix with a knife until the dough pulls away from the sides of the bowl. Slowly add water if the mixture seems too dry. Turn out onto a lightly floured surface and knead until smooth (about 3 minutes).

5. Place the dough in the prepared slow-cooker insert. Slice a cross on top of the dough and sprinkle the sesame seeds on top.

6. Cover and cook for 5–6 hours on low or 3 hours on high until the damper has cooked on the inside. Remove the damper by gently lifting up the sides of the baking paper. Set aside to cool slightly before slicing.

> **TRICKY TIP**
>
> You'll know the damper is cooked when it sounds hollow when tapped.

Variation: To make a sweet damper, omit the salt and dried herbs and replace with 2 tablespoons rice malt syrup and 1 teaspoon cinnamon (optional).

PROBIOTIC
GREEK YOGHURT

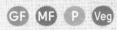

MAKES 1 litre

PREPARATION TIME
5 minutes

COOKING TIME
2½ hours on low
(+ 12 hours resting)

2 litres full-fat milk (preferably organic but not essential)

¾ cup (175 ml) full-fat organic, natural yoghurt with live cultures, at room temperature

1. Pour the milk into the slow-cooker insert. Cover and cook for 2½ hours on low. Allow the mixture to sit for 3 hours with the lid on.

2. Add the yoghurt, gently stir through the milk until well combined and replace the lid. Wrap a bath towel around the outside of the slow cooker, blocking out any light and keeping the cooker warm. Leave the yoghurt mixture in the slow cooker for 8–12 hours. This will produce runny yoghurt. Leave the yoghurt for an extra 4 hours if you'd like it to thicken further.

3. Line a strainer with cheesecloth or muslin. Place the strainer over a bowl (to catch the excess whey) then pour the mixture into the strainer and strain for at least one hour. Strain for longer if you want an even thicker yoghurt. Store in the fridge once desired consistency is reached.

> **TRICKY TIP**
>
> Freeze the whey in ice-cube trays and use for your next batch of yoghurt. Simply remove from the freezer and allow to return to room temperature before adding to yoghurt. Alternatively, add the whey to smoothies for a probiotic hit.

BUTTER-FREE PUMPKIN BUTTER

Use this veggie-packed butter as a spread on a slice of grain-free toast or Pumpkin and Zucchini Brekkie Pud (see page 142).

MAKES 1 cup (250 ml)

PREPARATION TIME
5 minutes

COOKING TIME
4 hours on low
2 hours on high

2 cups (500 ml) Pumpkin Purée

½ cup (125 ml) unsweetened almond milk (homemade or store-bought)

3 tablespoons rice malt syrup

½ teaspoon ground cinnamon

½ teaspoon ground nutmeg

½ teaspoon ground ginger

½ teaspoon sea salt

1. Combine the purée, almond milk and rice malt syrup in the slow-cooker insert. Add the spices and salt, stirring well.

2. Cover and cook for 4 hours on low or 2 hours on high. If the butter is too runny, remove the lid and cook for a further 30 minutes on high.

3. Scoop out into a container, cover and store in the fridge for up to 5 days. This butter is best served chilled.

TO MAKE PUMPKIN PURÉE

Preheat the oven to 200°C/gas 6. Peel and roughly chop 1 large pumpkin. Rub the pumpkin with olive oil and salt, and bake in the oven until tender, about 30–35 minutes. Allow to cool a little before blending in a food processor (or mash by hand) until smooth. Once completely cool, store separately in 1-cup (250 ml) batches in the freezer (in ziplock bags or containers).

HEARTY BREAKFASTS

*These slow-cooked breakfasts
have been designed to save you time
and help you start the day on
a nutritious note.*

ACTIVATED CACAO ZOATS

This is a super nutritious breakfast, loaded with hidden greens. The oats are soaked overnight to aid digestion. Soaking activates the enzymes in the oats, which help your body to break down the anti-nutrients and hard-to-digest components of the grain.

SERVES 6

PREPARATION TIME

1 minute
(+ 24 hours
soaking or
orvernight)

COOKING TIME

8 hours on low
4 hours on high

3 cups (300 g) rolled oats
(not the 'quick' variety)

2 litres water (or half-milk and
half-water, if you're not activating)

2 cups (450 g) grated courgettes

1 teaspoon sea salt

2 teaspoons ground cinnamon

2 tablespoons raw cacao powder

1½ teaspoons granulated stevia

nuts, nut butter, fresh berries, maca
powder, ground cinnamon, natural
yoghurt, or cacao nibs, to serve

THE MORNING BEFORE

1. To activate the oats, pour the oats and water into the slow-cooker insert. Allow to soak. Note: if you don't want to activate your oats skip this step and follow the instructions below.

THE NIGHT BEFORE

1. Combine all the ingredients in the slow-cooker insert. Cover and cook for 8 hours on low or 4 hours on high. if you activate your oats you will need to cook them for less time, approximately 5 hours on low or 2½ hours on high.

ON THE DAY

1. Stir the mixture. Spoon into bowls and top with your choice of topping.

CAVEMAN BREAKFAST MINCE

This brekkie option is great for anyone undergoing the 8-Week Programme. The combination of fats, greens and protein will stabilise blood sugar levels and help you avoid those sugary morning temptations.

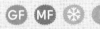

SERVES 6

PREPARATION TIME
5 minutes

COOKING TIME
8 hours on low
4 hours on high

800 g beef mince

1 onion, finely chopped

⅔ cup (100 g) frozen peas

2 tablespoons arrowroot
(if gluten-free or paleo) or cornflour,
mixed to a paste in cold water

2–3 garlic cloves,
chopped or crushed

1 cup (250 ml) Beginner's Beef Stock
(see page 26) (or store-bought
beef stock)

sea salt and freshly ground
black pepper, to taste

THE NIGHT BEFORE

1. Combine all the ingredients in the slow-cooker insert. Cover and cook for 8 hours on low or 4 hours on high.

THE NEXT MORNING

1. Stir the mince mixture and ladle out any excess liquid (save this for a soup base). Serve.

Suggested Sides:
- Wilted spinach cooked in coconut oil or butter
- Fried or poached eggs

MORNING TEA MUESLI SLICE

This has to be one of our favourite recipes. When we initially tested it, it was a dry stodgy brick but after experimenting with the recipe we managed to create a deceptively sweet 'n' gooey muesli slice that would happily please the masses at a morning tea.

SERVES 10–12

PREPARATION TIME
15 minutes

COOKING TIME
4 hours on low
2 hours on high

oil or butter, for greasing

½ cup (40 g) unsweetened shredded coconut

⅓ cup (45 g) almonds, roughly chopped

⅓ cup (40 g) walnuts, roughly chopped

¼ (30 g) cup pumpkin seeds

4 tablespoons white sesame seeds

1 cup (100 g) almond meal

1 egg, lightly beaten

½ cup (115 g) nut butter
(we prefer peanut or almond)

½ cup (100 g) coconut oil

½ cup (125 ml) rice malt syrup

1 teaspoon vanilla powder

cream, to serve (optional)

1. Grease the inside of the slow-cooker insert and line with baking paper so that it reaches halfway up the sides.

2. In a large bowl, combine the coconut, almonds, walnuts, pumpkin seeds and sesame seeds.

3. Add the almond meal and stir well before adding the egg and stirring well again.

4. In a saucepan, combine the nut butter, coconut oil, rice malt syrup and vanilla. Warm over low heat until the oil and rice malt syrup melt.

5. Stir the warmed mixture into the nut mixture and mix well. Press into the prepared slow-cooker insert.

6. Cover and cook for 4 hours on low or 2 hours on high. Once firm to the touch, switch off the slow cooker and allow to cool completely. Gently remove the slice by lifting up the sides of the baking paper. Slice into wedges and serve.

> **NOTE**
>
> The centre will be softer than the perimeter of the slice. If you want to cook it until firm, remove the lid and continue cooking for 30 minutes, or until you're happy with the consistency.

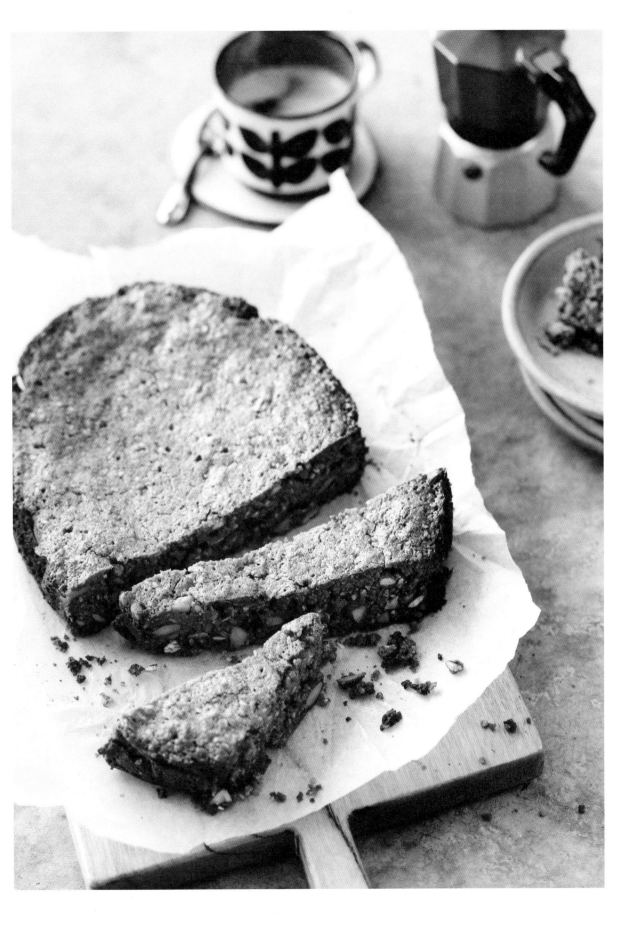

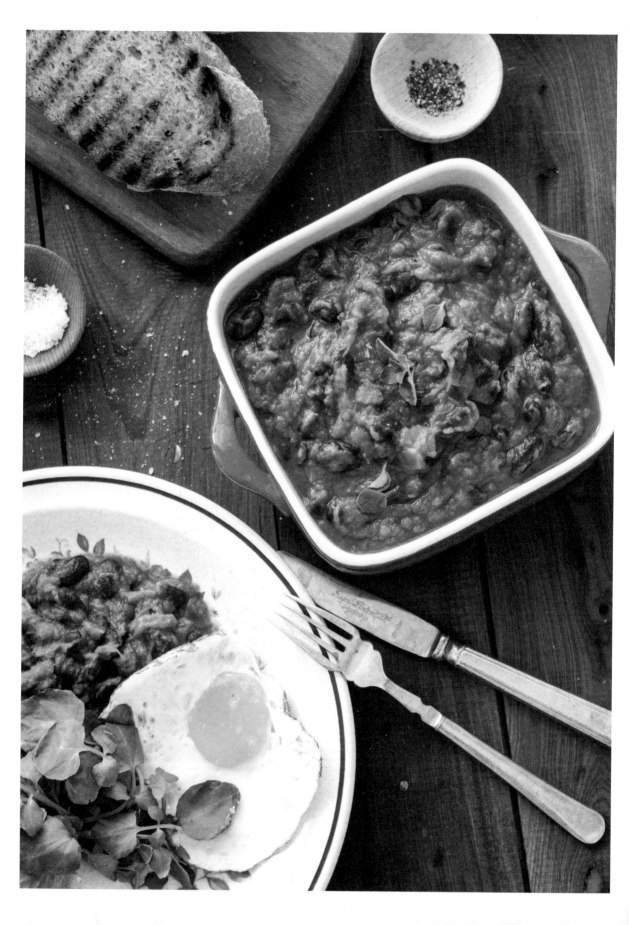

SWEET PUMPKIN
SUNDAY BEANS

These beans are deliciously sweet and way more appetising than the sugar-loaded varieties on shelves.

SERVES 6

PREPARATION TIME
5 minutes
(+ overnight
soaking)

COOKING TIME
6 hours on low
3 hours on high

2 cups (375 g) dried borlotti or kidney beans, soaked overnight (or 2 x 400 g cans, drained and rinsed)

300 g peeled pumpkin, chopped into 3 cm pieces

2 cups (500 ml) Chicken Stock (see page 28) (or store-bought chicken stock)

2 tablespoons sweet paprika

1 tablespoon dried oregano

½ teaspoon sea salt

1 teaspoon freshly ground black pepper

1. Rinse the soaked beans under cold running water, removing any discoloured ones, and toss into the slow cooker with the pumpkin.

2. Cover with the stock. Add the paprika, oregano, salt and pepper. Cover and cook for 6 hours on low or 3 hours on high or until the beans are soft.

3. Remove the lid and mash the pumpkin using a fork to thicken the sauce mixture.

TRICKY TIP

We like to make a big batch and freeze for the following week. It's great for mid-week lunches, too.

Suggested Sides:
- Fried or poached eggs
- Greens (watercress works well)
- Sourdough

PALEO VEGGIE FRITTATA

This is the perfect fridge-clean-out meal. Have a rummage through your fridge and use up any sad-looking veggies leftover from the week.

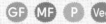

SERVES 6

PREPARATION TIME
5 minutes

COOKING TIME
5 hours on low
2½ hours on high

coconut oil, butter or ghee,
for greasing

10 eggs, whisked

1 cup (250 ml) milk (any type is fine)

1 red or green pepper, chopped

½ punnet cherry tomatoes

1 small onion, finely chopped

1 cup (50 g) spinach

75 g feta, crumbled

1 teaspoon sea salt

1 teaspoon freshly ground
black pepper

½ teaspoon dried cumin

½ teaspoon ground turmeric

½ cup (75 g) frozen peas

3 spring onions, finely chopped

fresh herbs, to serve

1. Grease the inside of the slow-cooker insert and line with baking paper so that it reaches halfway up the sides.

2. In a large bowl, combine the whisked eggs with the milk and then stir in the remaining ingredients.

3. Pour the frittata mixture into the prepared slow-cooker insert. Cover and cook for 5 hours on low or 2½ hours on high.

4. Once cooked, carefully remove the frittata by lifting up the sides of the baking paper.

5. Cut the frittata into slices and serve with fresh herbs. Store any remaining frittata in an airtight container in the fridge for up to three days.

TRICKY TIP

If you don't have a vegetable that's listed in the recipe, that's fine! Feel free to mix up the recipe with your favourite veggie combo.

SOUPS, STEWS AND CURRIES

*Winter warmers that are
great for the soul and packed with
immune-boosting goodness.*

VEGETABLE KORMA WITH QUINOA AND FLAKED ALMONDS

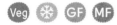

SERVES 6

PREPARATION TIME
10 minutes

COOKING TIME
8 hours on low
4 hours on high

½ head cauliflower, broken into florets

3 carrots, finely chopped

½ cup (125 ml) korma paste (look for sugar-free varieties)

½ cup (50 g) almond meal

1 onion, thinly sliced

2 garlic cloves, crushed

1 x 400 ml can coconut milk

1 cup (250 ml) Leftovers Vegetable Stock (see page 27) (or store-bought vegetable stock)

1 courgette, cut into chunks

1 red pepper, cut into 3 cm pieces

1 cup (70 g) washed and roughly chopped kale leaves

½ cup (75 g) frozen peas

2 baby yellow squash, quartered

3 cups (550 g) Cooked Quinoa (see below)

½ cup (50 g) flaked almonds, lightly toasted

fresh coriander leaves, to serve

1 cup (250 ml) Cucumber Raita (see page 116) or sliced cucumbers, to serve

IN THE MORNING

1. Combine the cauliflower, carrot, korma paste, almond meal, onion, garlic, coconut milk and stock in the slow-cooker insert. Cover and cook for 7½ hours on low or 3½ hours on high.

IN THE EVENING

1. Remove the lid and stir through the courgette, red pepper, kale, peas and squash. Cover and cook for another 30 minutes on high or until the vegetables have cooked through.

2. Serve the korma over a bed of warm quinoa and top with flaked almonds and coriander. Serve with Raita or sliced cucumber on the side.

COOKED QUINOA

Thoroughly rinse 2 cups (350 g) of quinoa. After rinsing, place the quinoa in a large saucepan and pour in 1 litre of water. Cover and bring to the boil, then reduce the heat and simmer, covered, for 15 minutes or until all the water has been absorbed. Remove the pan from the heat and let stand for 5 minutes, covered. Fluff the quinoa with a fork before serving.

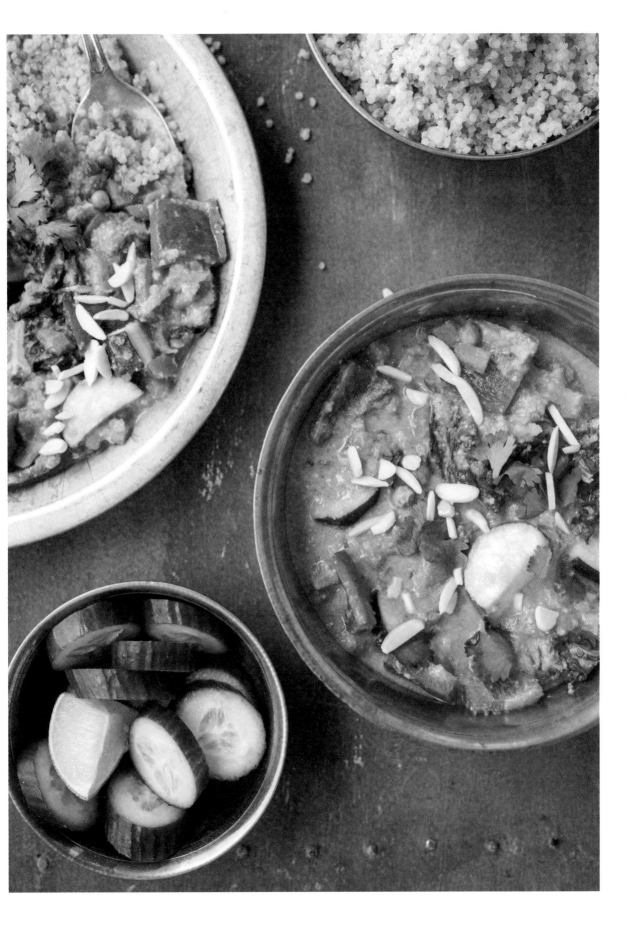

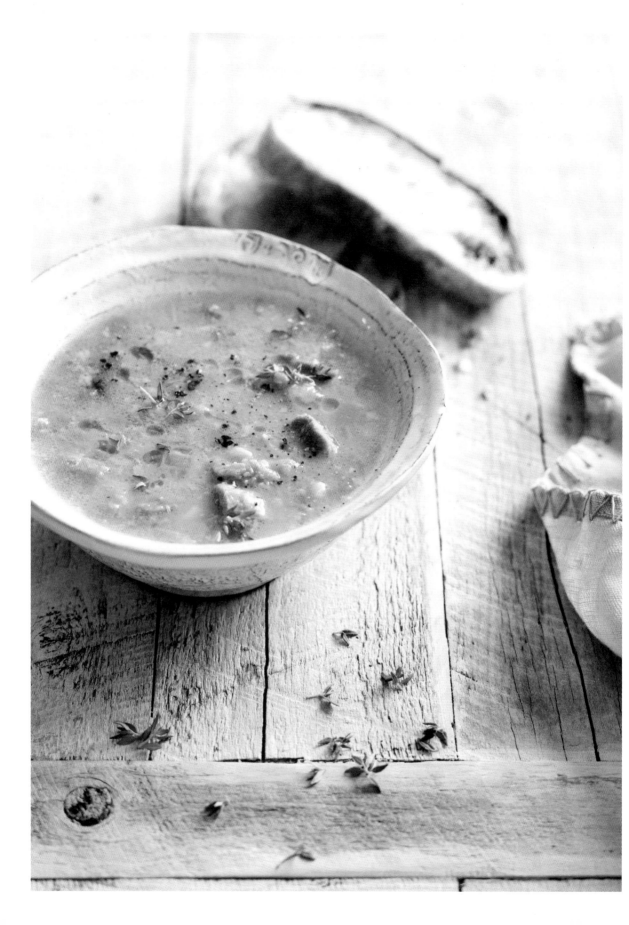

CLASSIC PEA
AND HAM SOUP

SERVES 6–8

PREPARATION TIME
10 minutes

COOKING TIME
8 hours on low
4 hours on high

500 g split peas, soaked
overnight and drained

2 litres water

1 ham hock (approx. 1.5 kg)

2 carrots, finely chopped

2 stalks celery, finely chopped

2 bay leaves

freshly ground black pepper,
to taste

2 tablespoons fresh thyme,
roughly chopped

IN THE MORNING

1. Place all the ingredients (except the thyme) in the slow-cooker insert. Cover and cook for 8 hours on low or 4 hours on high.

IN THE EVENING

1. Remove the bay leaves and the ham hock from the slow cooker. Pick off the meat from the bone and discard the bone. Use a stick blender to purée the soup to the desired consistency then stir back in the ham. Serve sprinkled with the fresh thyme.

TRICKY TIP

Because of the gelatinous nature of the ham hock your soup will solidify when cooled. Simply warm it up again in the slow cooker or over a low heat on the stovetop before serving.

Suggested Sides:
- Gluten-free Damper (see page 30) or toasted sourdough
- Natural, full-fat yoghurt or sour cream

THAI PUMPKIN 'N' CAULIFLOWER SOUP WITH PROBIOTIC GREEK YOGHURT

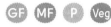

SERVES 6

PREPARATION TIME

10 minutes

COOKING TIME

8 hours on low
4 hours on high

2 potatoes, peeled, chopped into chunks

1 onion, finely chopped

2 garlic cloves, crushed

1 lemongrass stem, white part only, finely sliced

1 kaffir lime leaf, thinly sliced

2–3 cm knob ginger, skin removed, finely grated

1 teaspoon ground cumin

½ teaspoon ground turmeric

1–2 fresh red chillies, finely sliced (depending on how hot you like your soup)

½ head cauliflower, cut into small florets

500 g pumpkin or squash, chopped into chunks

sea salt and freshly ground black pepper, to taste

1.25 litres Leftovers Vegetable Stock (see page 27) (or store-bought vegetable stock)

½ (125 ml) cup Probiotic Greek Yoghurt (see page 31) (or natural full-fat yoghurt), to serve

fresh coriander leaves, to serve

IN THE MORNING

1. Place all the ingredients (saving some of the chilli to serve) except for the yoghurt and coriander in the slow-cooker insert. Cook for 8 hours on low or 4 hours on high.

IN THE EVENING

1. Use a stick blender to purée the ingredients to the desired consistency. Serve with a dollop of yoghurt, a sprinkle of coriander and sliced chilli.

Suggested Sides: •   Gluten-free Damper (see page 30) or toasted sourdough

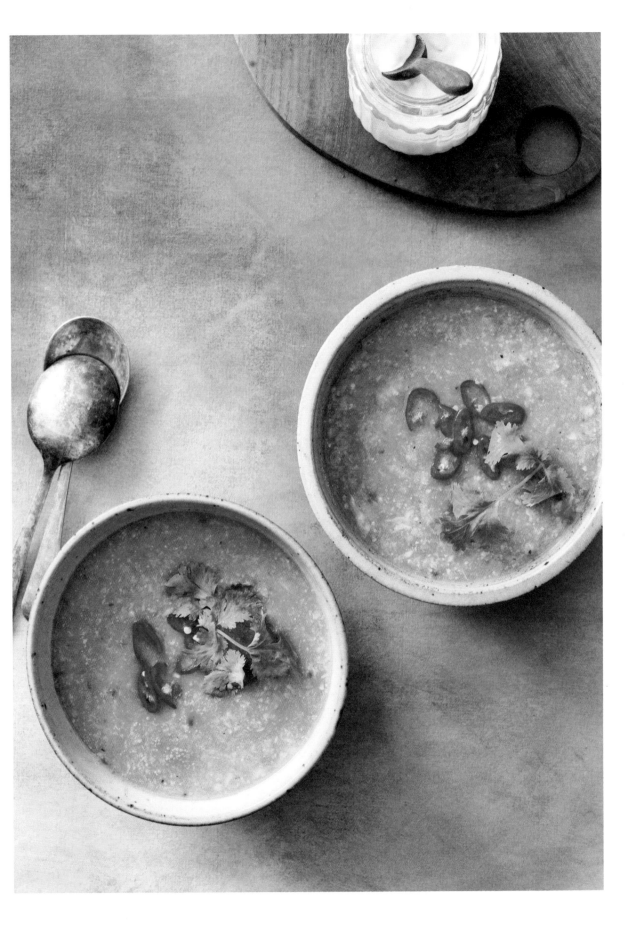

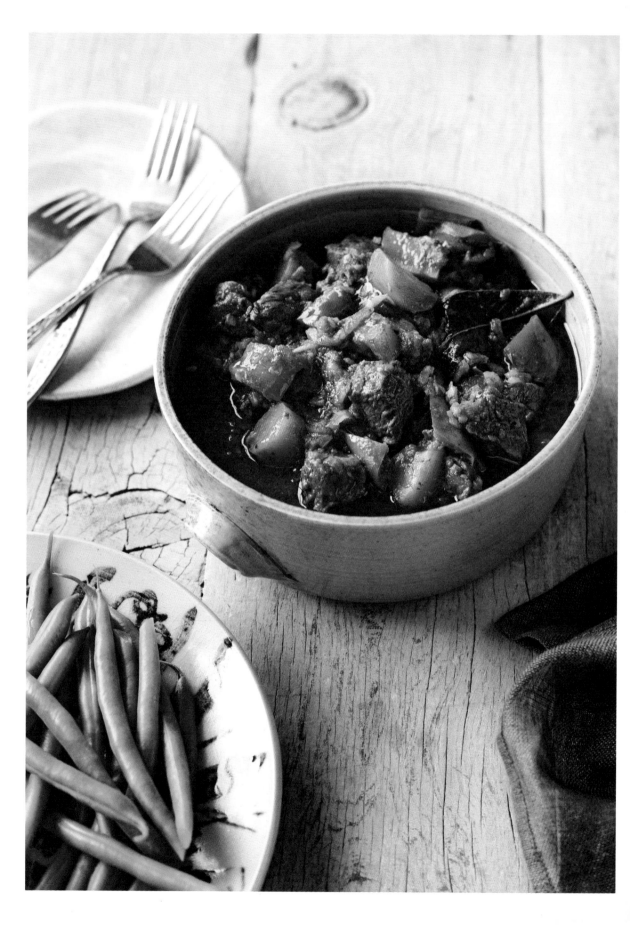

SARAH'S MUM'S HUNGARIAN GOULASH

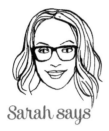

Sarah says

❝ This meal has very specific memories for me. Mum used to make it in a big cast-iron pot whenever we went camping. It was the meal we always ate the first night at the camp ground and it travelled there with us between Mum's feet in the front seat of the car. We'd arrive late, often in the dark, set up and then sit around on old milk crates with bowls of the stuff. Traditionally it's made with potatoes. I prefer substituting carrots, but feel free to do a combination of both. **❞**

SERVES 6

PREPARATION TIME
15 minutes

COOKING TIME
8 hours on low
4 hours on high

1 kg stewing beef (blade, chuck or brisket), cut into 2 cm cubes

4 carrots (or you can use 4 red potatoes), cut into 2 cm chunks

2 green peppers, cut into 2 cm chunks

3 tomatoes, peeled and quartered (approx. ½ x 400 g can chopped tomatoes)

2 onions, thinly sliced

2 tablespoons sweet paprika

2 tablespoons tomato purée

2 bay leaves

2 garlic cloves, crushed

1 teaspoon caraway seeds

½ teaspoon freshly ground black pepper

½ teaspoon sea salt

½ teaspoon granulated stevia (optional)

1 cup (250 ml) Beginner's Beef Stock (see page 26) (or store-bought beef stock)

fresh herbs, to serve

1. Place all the ingredients in the slow-cooker insert and stir to combine. Cover and cook for 8 hours on low or 4 hours on high. Serve sprinkled with fresh herbs.

Suggested Sides:
- Wholewheat pasta or rice or Thyme and Celeriac Mash (see page 132)
- Steamed greens

CHICKEN AND
WHITE BEAN SOUP

SERVES 6

PREPARATION TIME
5 minutes

COOKING TIME
8 hours on low
4 hours on high

600 g chicken thighs,
cut into chunks

1 onion, finely chopped

2 x 400 g cans cannellini beans,
rinsed and drained

2 carrots, peeled and finely chopped

2 stalks celery, finely chopped

1 teaspoon sea salt

½ teaspoon freshly ground
black pepper

1 garlic clove, crushed

2 tablespoons tomato purée

1 litre Chicken Stock (see page 28)
(or whatever stock you have)

2 tablespoons thyme leaves
(save some for garnishing)

1. Combine all the ingredients in the slow-cooker insert. Cover and cook
    for 8 hours on low or 4 hours for high. Sprinkle with fresh thyme
    before serving.

Suggested Sides: • Gluten-free Damper (see page 30)
                          or toasted sourdough

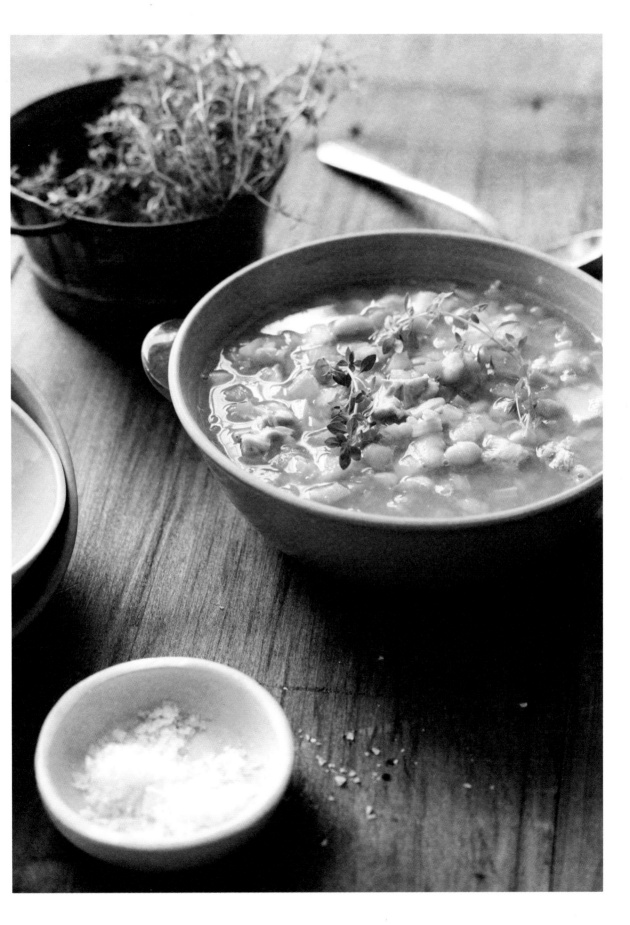

FRAGRANT MOROCCAN LAMB TAGINE

The kind of meal you'd skip a date with Ryan Gosling for . . .

SERVES 6

PREPARATION TIME
10 minutes
(+ overnight
marinating)

COOKING TIME
7 hours on low
3½ hours on high

1 teaspoon sweet paprika

1 teaspoon ground cumin

1 teaspoon ground turmeric

1 teaspoon ground cinnamon

1 teaspoon ground ginger

1.5 kg stewing lamb, diced

1 onion, finely sliced

1 tablespoon harissa paste

1 tablespoon tomato purée

2 cups (500 ml) Chicken Stock
(see page 28) (or store-bought
chicken stock)

½ x 400 g can chopped tomatoes

1 x 400 g can chickpeas, drained
and rinsed

½ cup (75 g) kalamata olives, pitted

½ cup (125 ml) Probiotic Greek Yoghurt
(see page 31) (or natural full-fat
yoghurt), to serve

½ cup (25 g) torn mint leaves

THE NIGHT BEFORE

1. In the slow-cooker insert, mix together all the dry spices and rub into the
   diced lamb, ensuring that the meat is covered. Cover and leave overnight
   in the fridge.

THE NEXT MORNING

1. In a bowl, combine the onion, harissa paste, tomato purée, stock and
   chopped tomatoes. Pour over the lamb and stir to combine. Cover and cook
   for 6 hours on low or 3 hours on high.

BEFORE SERVING

1. Lift off the lid and toss in the chickpeas and olives. Cover and cook for
   another hour on low or 30 minutes on high. Serve with a drizzle of yoghurt
   and torn mint leaves.

Suggested Sides:
- Cucumber Raita (see page 116) or sliced cucumbers
- Sweet Potato Mash (see page 132) or Cooked Quinoa
  (see page 42)

AUTUMNAL VEGGIE AND APPLE STEW

*This is a great recipe to try when you're slowly adding sweetness
back in during Week Six of the 8-Week Programme.*

SERVES 6

PREPARATION TIME

10 minutes

COOKING TIME

4 hours on low
2 hours on high

2 sweet potatoes, peeled and roughly chopped into chunks

200 g pumpkin or squash, cut into cubes

4 carrots, peeled and roughly chopped

4 parsnips, peeled and roughly chopped

1 onion, finely chopped

2 green apples, cored, peeled and roughly chopped

½ teaspoon sea salt

½ teaspoon freshly ground black pepper

½ teaspoon ground cumin

½ teaspoon ground cinnamon

3 cups (750 ml) Leftovers Vegetable Stock (see page 27) (or store-bought vegetable stock)

½ cup (25 g) flat-leaf parsley, roughly chopped

2 cups (150 g) roughly chopped Swiss chard

handful of pecans (optional), to serve

1. Place all the ingredients except the chard and pecans in the slow-cooker insert.

2. Cover and cook for 4 hours on low or 2 hours on high.

3. Add the chard and stir until wilted. Serve sprinkled with pecans.

> **TRICKY TIP**
>
> Use all the leftovers and offcuts from the vegetables in this dish to make more Leftovers Vegetable Stock (see page 27).

Suggested Sides:
- Gluten-free Damper (see page 30)
- Toasted sourdough

SPICED LAMB SHOULDER

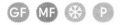

SERVES 6

PREPARATION TIME

10 minutes
(+ overnight
marinating)

COOKING TIME

8 hours on low
4 hours on high

1.5 cm knob ginger,
peeled and finely grated

6 large garlic cloves, crushed

1 tablespoon tomato purée

juice of ½ lime

2 teaspoons ground cumin

2 teaspoons smoked paprika

1 teaspoon ground coriander

1 teaspoon dried turmeric

1 teaspoon sumac

1 teaspoon chilli flakes

1 teaspoon sea salt

2 kg lamb shoulder, bone in

4 tablespoons olive oil

2 carrots, peeled and
roughly chopped

2 parsnips, peeled and
roughly chopped

1 red onion, peeled and
cut into wedges

1 sweet potato, peeled,
chopped into chunks

1½ cups (375 ml) water or Leftovers
Vegetable Stock (see page 27)
(or store-bought vegetable stock)

1 tablespoon arrowroot (if gluten-free
or paleo) or cornflour, mixed
to a paste in cold water

handful of coriander leaves,
chopped, to serve

THE NIGHT BEFORE

1. Combine the ginger, garlic, tomato purée, lime juice, spices and salt in a
   bowl. Score the lamb (2 cm deep) several times. Place the lamb in the slow-
   cooker insert. Drizzle with oil, and then rub on the spice mixture to coat,
   making sure to get into the grooves. Cover and place the slow-cooker insert
   in the fridge overnight to marinate.

IN THE MORNING

1. Tuck the veggies around the edges of the lamb and underneath if you
   need to. Pour water or stock into the slow-cooker insert. Cover and cook
   for 8 hours on low or 4 hours on high until the meat is tender and falling
   off the bone, taking care not to allow the slow cooker to run dry. Add
   ½ cup (125 ml) more water or stock to the slow cooker throughout cooking
   if the water has evaporated completely (remember to increase cooking
   time for 20–30 minutes each time if you do this).

IN THE EVENING

1. When cool enough to handle, transfer the lamb and veggies to a plate.
   Combine the cornflour mixture and stir into the sauce. Leave lid off and
   cook on high for 20 minutes or until the sauce thickens. Serve the veggies,
   lamb and gravy sprinkled with coriander.

Suggested Sides: •   Steamed greens

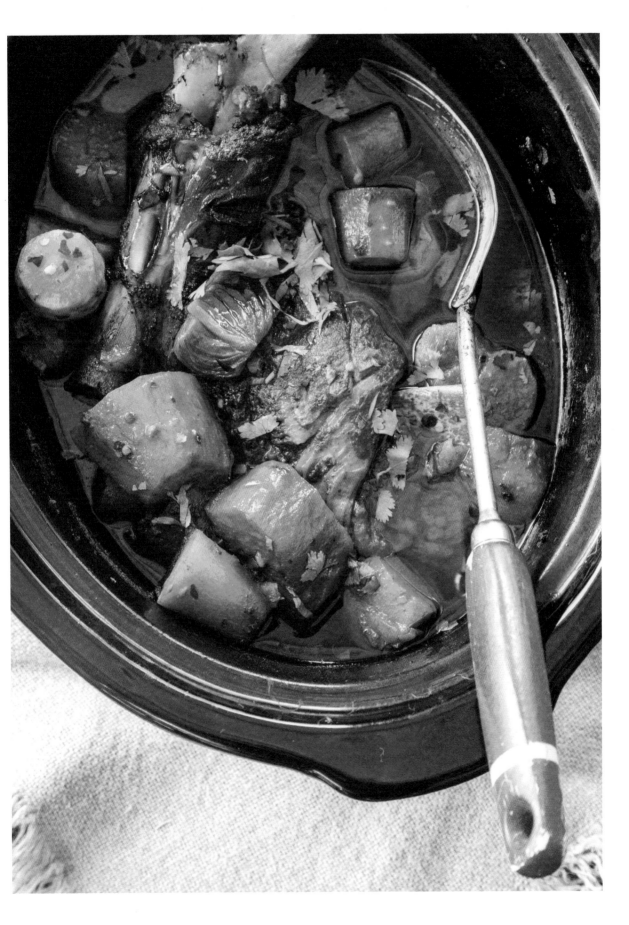

EASY BEEF CURRY

Renee shared her winning beef curry recipe. The pumpkin gives
wit an unexpected sweetness and makes it incredibly creamy.

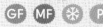

SERVES 6

PREPARATION TIME
5 minutes

COOKING TIME
7 hours on low
3½ hours on high

600 ml coconut milk

1 onion, finely chopped

2 garlic cloves, crushed

1 tablespoon ground cumin

1 tablespoon curry powder

**1–2 small red chillies, deseeded
and finely chopped**

600 g blade or chuck steak,

cut into small chunks

500 g pumpkin, chopped

**1 cup (about 150 g) chopped veggies
of your choice (courgettes and squash
work well)**

½ head cauliflower

½ cup (125 ml) natural full-fat yoghurt

fresh coriander leaves, to garnish

1. Pour the coconut milk into the slow-cooker insert. Add the onion, garlic,
   spices, chillies, beef and vegetables then stir well. Cover and cook for 7
   hours on low or 3½ hours on high. Serve with yoghurt, coriander and your
   choice of sides.

Suggested Sides:
- Basmati or jasmine rice
- Poppadoms
- Steamed greens
- Green salad

NAN'S COUNTRY CAPTAIN

Our book developer, Steph, shared this family recipe – it's her nan's signature dish. Country Captain originated in India and became a popular tinned meal, enjoyed by British officers during World War II. Her nan often used whatever ingredients she had spare to feed her brood of five.

SERVES 6

PREPARATION TIME
10 minutes

COOKING TIME
6 hours on low
3 hours on high

6 chicken thighs, cut into 3 cm chunks

1 onion, finely chopped

4 tablespoons desiccated coconut (optional)

3 garlic cloves, crushed

2 teaspoons curry powder

1 teaspoon ground turmeric

½ teaspoon cayenne pepper

1 cup (250 ml) coconut milk

½ cup (125 ml) Chicken Stock (see page 28) (or store-bought chicken stock)

1 tablespoon fish sauce

sea salt and freshly ground black pepper, to taste

½ cup (75 g) frozen peas or mangetout

IN THE MORNING

1. Place the chicken, onion, coconut, garlic, spices, coconut milk, stock and fish sauce in the slow-cooker insert. Season with salt and pepper and stir until combined. Cover and cook for 6 hours on low or 3 hours on high.

IN THE EVENING

2. Remove the lid and add the peas or mangetout. If the curry looks like it has reduced too much add some extra stock. Cover and cook on high for a further 10 minutes until the peas or mangetout are cooked. Serve.

Suggested Sides:
- Basmati rice or jasmine rice
- Lime wedges
- Fresh coriander leaves
- Flaked almonds

THAI GREEN
CURRY 'N' SQUASH

Spaghetti squash (also known as vegetable spaghetti) is a staple in American fruit and veg stores. You can find it in some stores in Australia and Europe as well. This clever veggie, once cooked, can be shredded into pasta-like strands and makes a nice substitute for wheat pasta. The beauty of this dish is you cook your 'pasta' with the curry — a one-pot miracle!

SERVES 6

PREPARATION TIME
5 minutes

COOKING TIME
4½ hours on low
2½ hours on high

1 spaghetti squash

2 tablespoons green curry paste
(opt for sugar-free/low-sugar varieties)

2 x 400 ml cans full-fat coconut milk,
at room temperature

4 tablespoons water

½ head cauliflower, cut into florets

2 cups (225 g) mangetout or green
beans, trimmed

2 courgettes, chopped into chunks

fresh coriander leaves, to serve

1. Cut the spaghetti squash in half widthways. Scoop out the seeds — they are delicious roasted.

2. Using a fork, poke holes into the tops of the squash halves.

3. Combine the curry paste, coconut milk and water in the slow-cooker insert. Mix well.

4. Place the spaghetti squash halves, cut-side down, into the coconut curry mixture. Add the cauliflower. Cover and cook for 4 hours on low or 2 hours on high.

BEFORE SERVING

1. Toss in the mangetout or beans and courgettes. Use a spoon to baste the vegetables with the coconut mixture. Cover and cook on low for a further 30 minutes.

2. Carefully (they'll be hot!) remove the squash halves from your slow cooker. Once cool enough to handle, using tongs and a fork, scrape the squash in spaghetti-like strands into serving bowls.

3. Ladle the sauce and vegetables over the spaghetti squash. Serve sprinkled with the coriander.

TRICKY TIP

If you can't find spaghetti squash, add extra courgettes and baby yellow squash during Step 4 instead.

Suggested Sides:
- Steamed Asian greens
- Jasmine rice or Cooked Quinoa (see page 42)

WEEKDAY DUMP 'N' RUN

*Simply throw the ingredients
into the slow cooker and press play.
Come home to a ready-made dinner
without all the fuss!*

SARAH'S CINNAMON BEEF CHEEKS

SERVES 6

PREPARATION TIME
5 minutes

COOKING TIME
8 hours on low
4 hours on high

4–5 beef cheeks (approx. 1 kg), fat trimmed, each cheek cut into 2–3 even-sized pieces

1 tablespoon olive oil

200 g portobello mushrooms (or any mushrooms), roughly chopped

1 carrot, roughly chopped

2 stalks celery, roughly chopped

1 onion, finely chopped

2 garlic cloves, crushed

3 bay leaves

1 teaspoon thyme leaves, roughly chopped

1 teaspoon rosemary leaves, roughly chopped

2 teaspoons ground cinnamon or 2 cinnamon sticks

1 teaspoon vanilla powder (optional)

1 tablespoon tomato purée (optional)

1 cup (250 ml) Beginner's Beef Stock (see page 26) (or store-bought beef stock)

¾ cup (175 ml) dry sherry, such as Pedro Ximenez (or red wine; or a combo of both)

1 tablespoon arrowroot (if gluten-free) or cornflour, mixed to a paste in cold water (optional)

IN THE MORNING

1. Place the beef cheeks in the slow-cooker insert. Place the rest of the ingredients (except the arrowroot or cornflour) on top in the order listed. Cover and cook for 8 hours on low or 4 hours on high or until the meat is tender and falls apart easily.

IN THE EVENING

1. If you like a thicker sauce, pour the arrowroot or cornflour paste into the slow-cooker insert, stir and cook for 30 minutes on high with the lid off. Serve with your choice of sides.

Suggested Sides:
- Cooked Quinoa (see page 42) or jasmine rice
- Steamed green beans

ONE-POT APPLE CIDER CHICKEN

SERVES 6

PREPARATION TIME
5 minutes

COOKING TIME
6 hours on low
3 hours on high

1 kg bone-in chicken thighs

2 spring onions, thinly sliced

2 bay leaves

2–3 garlic cloves, crushed

4 tablespoons tamari or soy sauce

4 tablespoons apple cider vinegar

juice of ½ lemon

2 tablespoons chopped flat-leaf parsley

1. Place the chicken in the slow-cooker insert. Combine all the other ingredients in a small bowl. Pour over the chicken and toss lightly to coat.

2. Cover and cook for 6 hours on low or 3 hours on high.

3. Remove the bones from the slow cooker leaving the chicken behind. Save the bones to make Chicken Stock (see page 28) later. Shred the chicken and ladle the sauce over the meat once dished up. Serve sprinkled with more parsley.

Suggested Sides: • Steamed green beans or tenderstem broccoli

• Cooked Quinoa (see page 42)

ICARIAN LEMON PORK

My travels with National Geographic in the world's Blue Zones (where people live longest) dug up this surprising fact: the one meat all 'zones' have in common is pork. In Icaria, a Greek island and one of the five zones, this kind of dish is very typical.

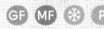

SERVES 6

PREPARATION TIME
5 minutes

COOKING TIME
8½ hours on low
4½ hours on high

1 kg pork, preferably shoulder, cut into cubes, or about 6 pork chops (some fat removed)

4 tablespoons stock or water (any type will work)

juice of 2 lemons

⅓ cup (75 ml) olive oil

1 onion, sliced into rings

2 garlic cloves, crushed

sea salt

1–2 tablespoons arrowroot (if gluten-free or paleo) or cornflour

IN THE MORNING

1. Place the pork in the slow-cooker insert and pour the stock or water, half of the lemon juice and the oil over the top. Place the onion and garlic on top. Sprinkle with plenty of salt. Cover and cook for 8 hours on low or 4 hours on high.

IN THE EVENING

1. Ladle out some of the juices, mix with a tablespoon or two of arrowroot or cornflour and the rest of the lemon juice. Pour back over the meat and stir. Cover and cook for another 30 minutes.

Suggested Sides:
- Cooked Quinoa (see page 42) or Thyme and Celeriac Mash (see page 132)
- Steamed greens or Greek salad
- Olives and feta cheese

PESTO CHICKEN WITH GREEN OLIVES AND QUINOA

We've made this recipe as simple as possible. Even the quinoa is cooked in the same pot!

SERVES 6

PREPARATION TIME
5 minutes (+ 10 mins standing)

COOKING TIME
7½ hours on low
4 hours on high

1 aubergine, cut into 3 cm cubes

½ cup (75 g) pitted green olives

1 x 400 g can chickpeas, rinsed and drained

3 tablespoons homemade basil pesto (or store-bought pesto)

1 teaspoon ground cumin

1 teaspoon ground coriander

1 teaspoon dried oregano

½ teaspoon sea salt

freshly ground black pepper

6 chicken thigh fillets or drumsticks

2 cups (500 ml) Chicken Stock (see page 28) (or store-bought chicken stock)

1 cup (170 g) uncooked quinoa, rinsed twice

IN THE MORNING

1. Place the aubergine, olives, chickpeas and pesto in the slow-cooker insert. Sprinkle with the spices and salt and pepper. Lay the chicken thighs on the top of the mixture. Stir to coat the chicken with the seasoning. Pour the stock over all the ingredients.

2. Cover and cook for 7 hours on low or 3½ hours on high or until the chicken is cooked through and tender.

IN THE EVENING

1. Remove the chicken from the slow cooker and pour in the rinsed quinoa. Stir well. Return the chicken to the slow cooker.

2. Cover again and cook for 20–30 minutes on high or until the quinoa is cooked (it should have 'tails' sprouting). Turn off the slow cooker, remove the lid and allow to sit for 10 minutes before serving.

GROUNDING BEEF
AND ROOTS STEW

*I often talk about Ayurvedic healing, which focuses on correcting imbalances.
For anyone who finds themselves agitated, anxious or 'brittle', this recipe is fabulous –
hearty meat dishes and root veggies are best for you.*

SERVES 6

PREPARATION TIME
10 minutes

COOKING TIME
8½ hours on low
4½ hours on high

500 g chuck steak,
cut into large cubes

½ teaspoon sea salt

freshly ground black pepper

1 onion, cut into wedges

2 garlic cloves, crushed

2½ cups (600 ml) Chicken Stock (see
page 28) (or store-bought chicken
stock)

½ cup (125 ml) red wine

extra water, if required

2 carrots, halved and cut into
quarters lengthways

2 parsnips, halved and cut into
quarters lengthways

1 large swede, cut into wedges

flat-leaf parsley, chopped, to serve

IN THE MORNING

1. Place the beef in the slow-cooker insert and season with salt and pepper.
   Add the onion, garlic, stock and red wine. Cover and cook for 7½ hours on
   low or 3½ hours on high.

BEFORE SERVING

1. If the meat looks like it's drying out add ¼–½ cup (60–120 ml) extra water or
   stock. Add the vegetables. Cover and cook for 1 hour on high or until the
   vegetables are tender when pricked with a fork. Serve the meat
   and root veggies sprinkled with parsley.

Suggested Sides: • Steamed green beans or other greens

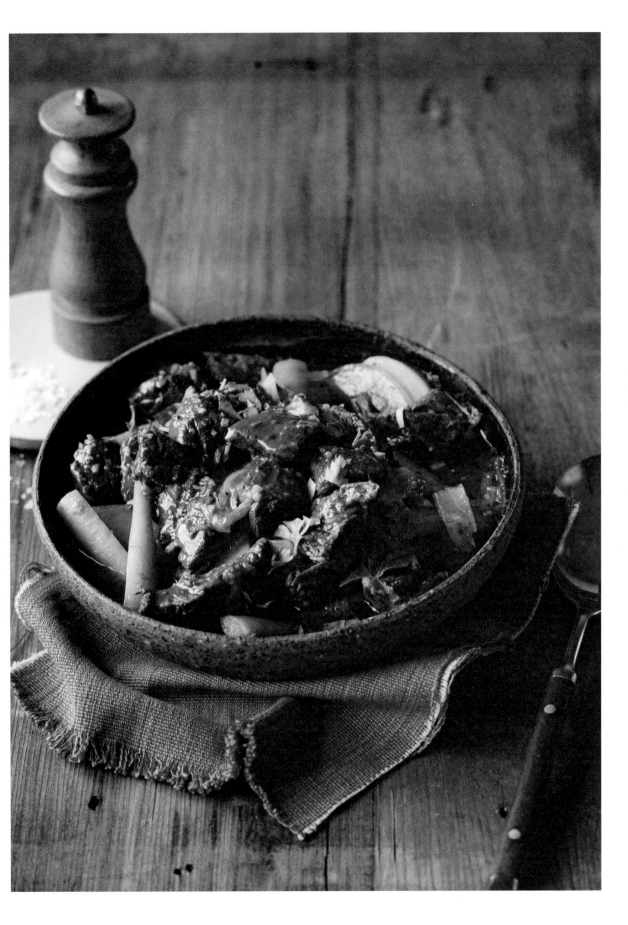

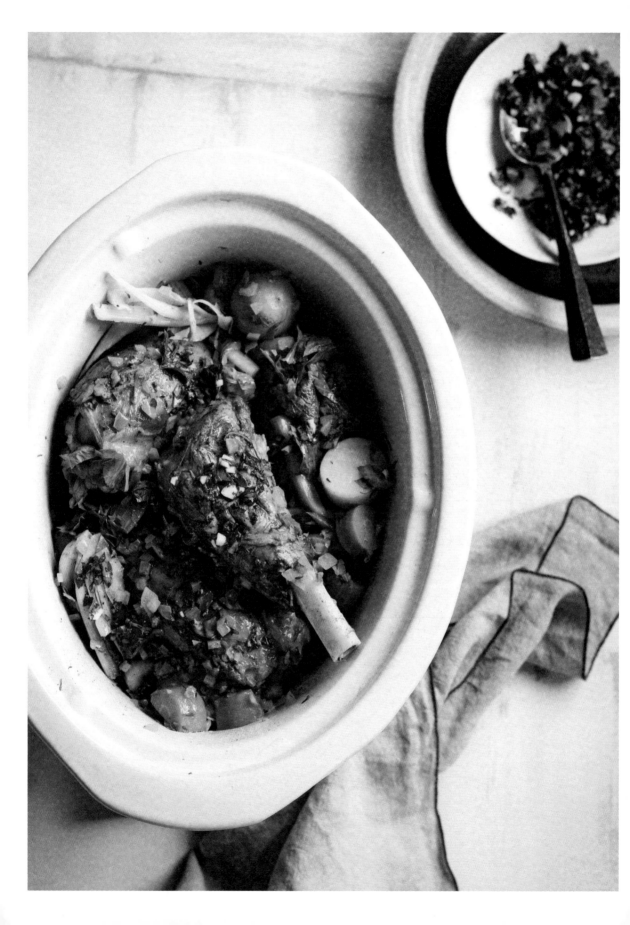

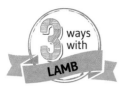

1. LEMON AND CINNAMON LAMB SHANKS WITH A LEMONY GREMOLATA

Cooking lamb shanks slowly allows you to separate the meat easily from the bone.
Use any leftover lamb in this dish to make two more delicious meals.

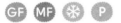

SERVES 6–8

PREPARATION TIME
10 minutes

COOKING TIME
8 hours on low
4 hours on high

1 large onion, finely chopped

1 large carrot, chopped into 2 cm chunks

1 small fennel bulb, sliced into 1.5 cm wedges (reserve fronds for later)

3 stalks celery, chopped into 2 cm chunks (reserve the leaves, chopped)

200 g baby new potatoes, halved

4–6 lamb shanks (approx. 1.5 kg)

2 garlic cloves, crushed

1 cup (250 ml) Chicken Stock (see page 28) (or store-bought chicken stock)

½ cup (125 ml) white wine or extra chicken stock

dash of apple cider vinegar

1 bay leaf

1 teaspoon dried thyme

1 teaspoon ground cinnamon

1 tablespoon chopped preserved lemon or juice of 2 lemons

LEMONY GREMOLATA

¾ bunch flat-leaf parsley, very finely chopped

6–8 garlic cloves, very finely chopped

grated zest and juice of 2 lemons or 2 tablespoons chopped preserved lemon

4 tablespoons extra virgin olive oil

1 teaspoon sea salt

IN THE MORNING

1. Place the onion, carrot, fennel, celery and potatoes in the slow-cooker insert. Arrange the shanks on top then add the remaining ingredients (except fennel fronds, celery leaves and Lemony Gremolata) over the lot. Stir a little (no need to mix completely). Cover and cook for 8 hours on low or 4 hours on high.

BEFORE SERVING

1. In the final 20 minutes, add the fennel fronds and celery leaves. To make the Lemony Gremolata, combine all the ingredients in a jar and shake vigorously.

2. Once you're ready to serve, remove the shanks and pull the meat from the bones. Serve with the Lemony Gremolata.

Suggested Sides: • Steamed tenderstem broccoli or other steamed greens

• Sweet Potato Mash (see page 132)

2. SHANKY SHEPHERD'S PIE

Okay, so this isn't a slow-cooker recipe as such, but is a great way to serve up your shanks.

SERVES 4–6

PREPARATION TIME
10 minutes

COOKING TIME
40 minutes

2 teaspoons coconut oil, butter or ghee

4 small carrots, finely chopped

2 onions, finely chopped

1 teaspoon ground cumin

3–4 portions cooked lamb shanks, shredded or 500 g stewed lamb meat

1 x 400 g can brown lentils, drained and rinsed

½ cup (125 ml) Chicken Stock (see page 28) (or other stock if you prefer)

2 cups (500 ml) Sweet Potato Mash (see page 132)

80 g butter

1. Preheat the oven to 200°C/gas 6.

2. In a large pot or saucepan, heat the oil and sauté the carrots, onion and cumin until soft and fragrant. Add the shredded meat, lentils and stock and simmer for 2–3 minutes.

3. Spoon the mixture into a lightly greased pie dish, or 4–6 individual pie ramekins, and spread the Sweet Potato Mash over the top.

4. Dot with the butter and bake for about 25 minutes, or until golden.

Suggested Sides:
- Steamed courgettes
- Mangetout

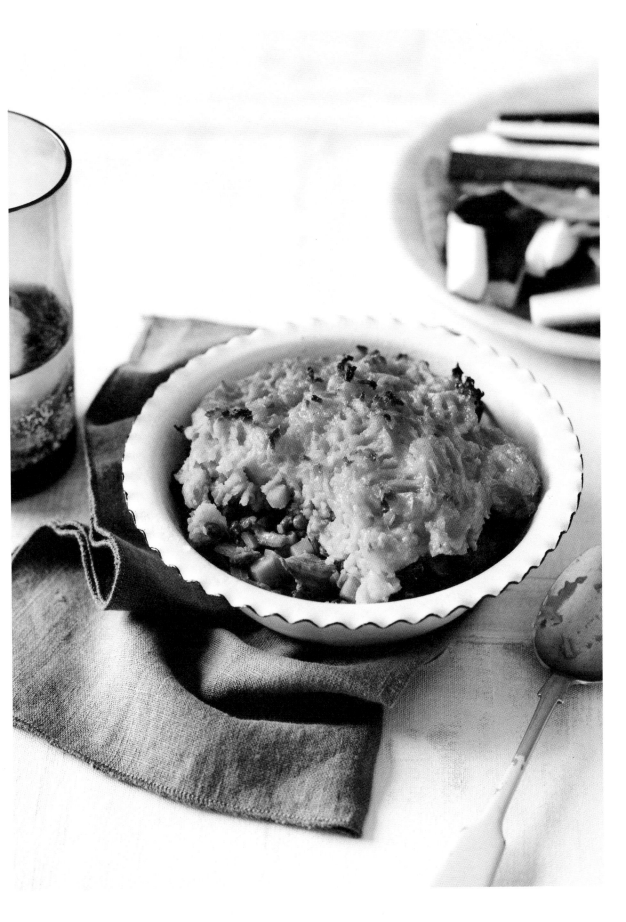

3. SPICED LAMB AND CHICKPEA STEW

GF MF ❄

SERVES 4–6

PREPARATION TIME
10 minutes

COOKING TIME
6 hours on low
3 hours on high

500 g lamb stewing meat or
3–4 portions leftover lamb shanks

600 g pumpkin or squash, peeled
and cut into cubes

2 courgettes, cut into 2 cm pieces

1 x 400 g can chickpeas,
drained and rinsed

2 carrots, chopped

1 onion, chopped

2 stalks celery, chopped

2 garlic cloves, crushed

2 tablespoons ground cumin

1 tablespoon harissa paste

1 tablespoon smoked paprika

1 litre Chicken Stock (see page 28)
(or store-bought chicken stock)

½ x 400 g can chopped tomatoes

1 tablespoon arrowroot (if gluten-free
or paleo) or cornflour, mixed to a paste
in cold water

flat-leaf parsley, to serve

1. Combine all the ingredients in the slow-cooker insert (if using uncooked stewing meat, add it in now), except the leftover lamb and arrowroot or cornflour paste. Cover and cook for 5 hours on low or 2½ hours on high or until the vegetables are tender and the stew base has reduced. If the stew doesn't look thick enough, add in the arrowroot or cornflour paste. Mix well.

2. Remove the lid and stir in the leftover lamb, if using. Cover and continue cooking for 1 hour on low or 30 minutes on high.

3. Ladle into bowls and serve sprinkled with parsley.

Suggested Sides: • Gluten-free Damper (see page 30)
or Cooked Quinoa (see page 42)

COMFORT CLASSICS

A chapter of our favourite home-style
recipes inspired by wintery weekends
and Sunday pot-roasts.

CHEAT'S BANGERS 'N' MASH

You can buy a pre-packaged bag of diced carrot, celery and onion at your local supermarket to make this recipe a super easy, mid-week meal. The best part? The potatoes collapse all by themselves so no mashing required!

SERVES 6

PREPARATION TIME
5 minutes

COOKING TIME
8 hours on low
4 hours on high

4 potatoes, peeled, washed and cut into chunks

2 onions, sliced into rings

1 cup (150 g) roughly chopped carrot

1 cup (100 g) roughly chopped celery

8 thick sausages (pork or beef), cut into thirds

1 tablespoon garlic powder or garlic clove

1 teaspoon sea salt

1 teaspoon freshly ground black pepper

1 cup (250 ml) Beginner's Beef Stock (see page 26) (or store-bought beef stock)

IN THE MORNING

1. Place the potato, onion, carrot, celery and then sausages in the slow-cooker insert. Add the garlic and season with salt and pepper. Stir gently to combine and pour the stock evenly over the top. Cover and cook for 8 hours on low or 4 hours on high.

IN THE EVENING

1. Remove the sausages from the slow-cooker insert and use a fork to mash any chunks of potato to the desired consistency. Serve the sausages and mash with your choice of sides.

Suggested Sides:
- Cider-glazed Beets (see page 124) or Easy Slaw (see page 97)
- Steamed greens

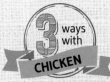

1. ROAST CHOOK WITH LEEKS AND FENNEL

Roasting a whole bird is the most economical way to eat chicken. Use this recipe as a base to cook Sarah's Mum's Chicken Soup (see page 74) and Mexican Chilli Chicken Tacos (see page 77). You'll need some kitchen string for this recipe.

SERVES 6

PREPARATION TIME
15 minutes

COOKING TIME
6 hours on low
3 hours on high

1.5 kg whole organic chicken

1 lemon, unpeeled, roughly chopped

5 garlic cloves, unpeeled, smashed with the back of your knife

5 fresh thyme sprigs

5 stems flat-leaf parsley

100 g butter

2 baby fennel bulbs or 1 medium fennel bulb

1 leek

⅔ cup (150 ml) white wine

2 bay leaves

1 cup (250 ml) Chicken Stock (see page 28) (or store-bought chicken stock, or water)

2–3 tablespoons arrowroot (if gluten-free) or cornflour, mixed to a paste in cold water

IN THE MORNING

1. Wash the chicken and pat dry. Stuff with the lemon, garlic and herbs. No need to be delicate. Tie the legs with kitchen string.

2. Melt the butter in a hot frying pan and brown the bird all over. Meanwhile, remove some of the fronds and woody ends from the fennel and cut bulb lengthways into 2 cm wedges and place in the slow-cooker insert.

3. Remove the dark green ends of the leek, cut the remainder into 2 x 15 cm (roughly) lengths, then slice each lengthwise in four. Add to the fennel. Place the chicken on top.

4. Add wine to the frying pan and bring to the boil. Pour the wine over the chicken and vegetables, setting aside the pan for later. Add the bay leaf and stock and cover with the lid. Cook 6 hours on low or 3 hours on high.

BEFORE SERVING

1. To make the gravy, drain the juices from the slow cooker into the reserved frying pan and bring to a simmer, adding the arrowroot paste. Stir until it thickens.

Suggested Sides:
- Garden salad or steamed tenderstem broccoli
- Sweet Potato Mash (see page 132)

2. SARAH'S MUM'S CHICKEN SOUP

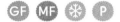

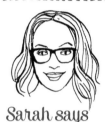

Sarah says

" This recipe is wonderfully evocative for me. In winter, Mum would always put a big pot of stock on the stove on Saturday and it would bubble away for hours, then Sunday lunch was chicken soup full of root vegetables and herbs. "

SERVES 4–6

PREPARATION TIME
5 minutes

COOKING TIME
4 hours on low
2 hours on high

2 carrots, cut into 1.5 cm slices

1 onion, roughly chopped

1 stalk celery, cut into 1.5 cm slices, leaves roughly chopped

1 swede or turnip, cut into 1.5 cm slices

2 courgettes, cut into 1.5 cm slices

2 tablespoons seaweed (optional)

handful of flat-leaf parsley, chopped

3–4 portions leftover shredded chicken or 400 g diced chicken thighs (if you don't have leftovers)

1.5 litres Chicken Stock (see page 28) (or store-bought chicken stock)

1. Add the carrot, onion, celery, swede or turnip, courgettes, seaweed (if using), parsley and stock to the slow-cooker insert. Add the diced chicken thigh, if using, and stir to combine. Cover and cook for 4 hours on low or 2 hours on high.

BEFORE SERVING

1. If you're using the leftover chicken remove the lid 30 minutes before serving and add to the slow cooker to heat through.

Suggested Sides: • Ham and cheese toasted sandwiches

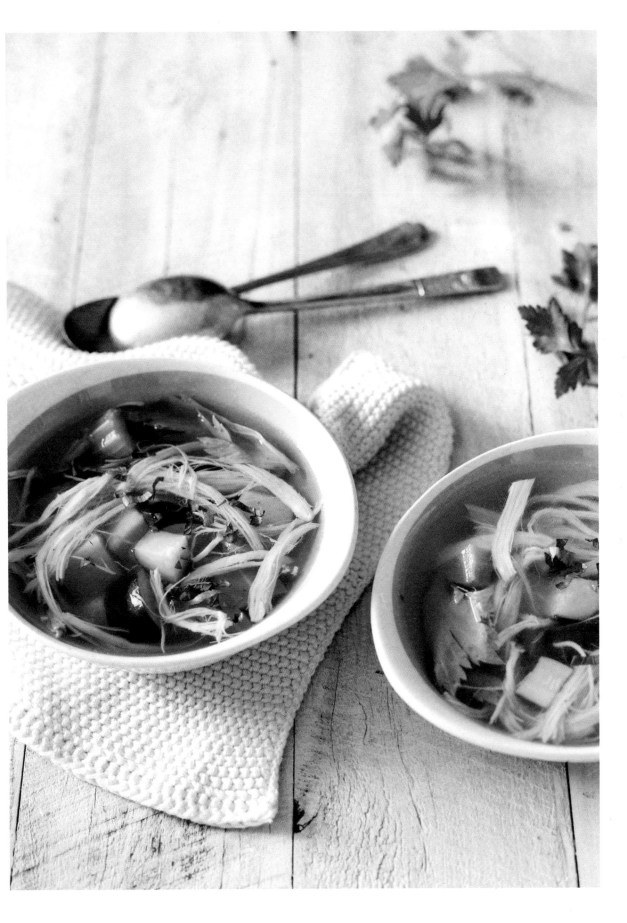

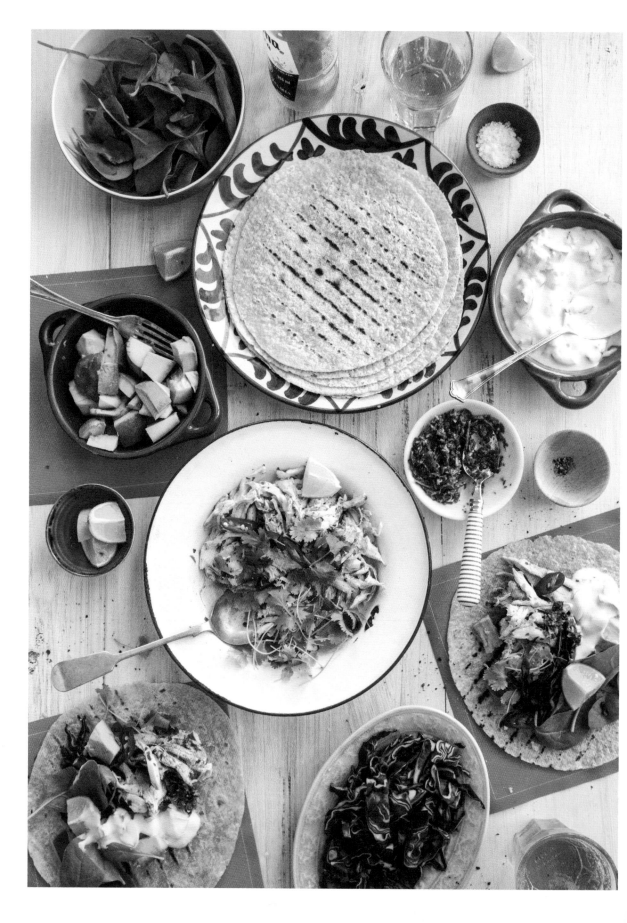

3. MEXICAN CHILLI CHICKEN TACOS

This recipe came about organically at our photo shoot. We had all this delicious food and the natural decision was to do a bit of a 'make-your-own taco' spread for lunch. If you don't have leftover chicken you can use 500 g chicken mince or half a roast chicken from the supermarket instead (it tastes just as good).

SERVES 4–6

PREPARATION TIME
5 minutes

COOKING TIME
1½ hours on low
45 minutes on high

3–4 portions leftover chicken, shredded (or whatever amount you have) or 500 g chicken mince

4 tablespoons Chicken Stock (see page 28) (or store-bought chicken stock)

1 onion, finely sliced

4 garlic cloves, crushed

juice of 2 limes

1 tablespoon olive oil

1 teaspoon ground cumin

1 teaspoon chilli powder

1 teaspoon smoked paprika

sea salt and freshly ground black pepper, to taste

1 red chilli, sliced with seeds (optional)

1 cup (30 g) fresh coriander leaves, roughly chopped

6 small gluten-free tortillas

TOPPINGS

¼ red cabbage, shredded

1 avocado, mashed or cubed

fresh coriander leaves

lime wedges

sour cream

Cucumber Raita (see page 116) or tzatziki

Lemony Gremolata (see page 67)

1. Place the shredded chicken (or mince) in the slow-cooker insert. Add the stock, onion, garlic, lime juice, olive oil, spices and salt and pepper. Stir all the ingredients to ensure the chicken is coated.

2. Cover and cook for 1½ hours on low or 45 minutes on high. Once cooked, scatter with chilli and coriander. Warm the tortillas in the microwave or grill. Serve the chilli chicken mixture, tortillas and toppings separately. Let everyone help themselves.

MATT PRESTON'S SLOW-ROASTED PORK SHOULDER WITH APPLE AND LEEKS

Matt Preston is the king of the traditional hearty roast. He kindly let us adapt this recipe from his book Fast, Fresh and Unbelievably Delicious *for a slow cooker.*

SERVES 6–8

PREPARATION TIME
10 minutes

COOKING TIME
8 hours on low
4½ hours on high

1.25 kg pork shoulder, boned and rolled, fat removed (ask the butcher to do this for you)

1 teaspoon sea salt

APPLE AND LEEKS

3 tablespoons olive oil

3 tablespoons cider

1 tablespoon rice malt syrup

1 tablespoon sage leaves, finely chopped

2 large leeks, cut in half lengthways and then into 5 cm pieces

1½–2 green apples, peeled, cored and cut into wedges

sea salt and freshly ground black pepper

CIDER GRAVY

⅔ cup (150 ml) cider

1 cup (250 ml) Chicken Stock (see page 28) (or store-bought chicken stock)

1 tablespoon rice malt syrup

1 garlic clove, crushed

½ onion, finely sliced

sea salt and freshly ground black pepper, to taste

30 g butter

1 tablespoon sage leaves, finely chopped

IN THE MORNING

1. Score the skin of the pork and season with sea salt. Place the pork in the slow-cooker insert. Cover and cook for 7 hours on low or 3½ hours on high.

IN THE EVENING

1. To prepare the apple and leek mixture, whisk together the oil, cider and rice malt syrup. Add the chopped sage. Coat the leeks and apple with the cider dressing, and season with salt and pepper.

2. Remove the lid of the slow cooker. Add the apples and leeks around the side of the pork. Cover and cook for another hour on high until the leeks are tender.

BEFORE SERVING

1. To make the cider gravy, first remove the pork, apple and leeks from the slow-cooker insert. Cover with foil to keep warm. Turn the slow cooker to high. Add the cider, chicken stock, syrup, garlic and onion and stir. Season with salt and pepper. Leave, uncovered, until the mixture has thickened to a gravy, then whisk in the butter and add the sage.

2. Carve the pork and serve with the apple, leeks and gravy.

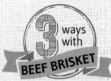

ways with
BEEF BRISKET

1. BEEF POT ROAST WITH BRAISED COCO-NUTTY CABBAGE

Use the leftover beef from your pot roast to make a batch of Hearty Irish Beef Stew and a warming bowl of Beef Hash (see page 80).

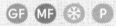

SERVES 6

PREPARATION TIME
10 minutes

COOKING TIME
8–10 hours on low
4–5 hours on high

3 large parsnips, peeled and cut into large chunks

3 carrots, ends trimmed (use in the Leftovers Vegetable Stock; see page 27) and chopped into thirds

2 onions, quartered

800 g whole beef topside, brisket or blade roast

sea salt and freshly ground black pepper, to taste

3 fresh rosemary sprigs

5 garlic cloves, crushed

½ cup (125 ml) Beginner's Beef Stock (see page 26) (or store-bought beef stock)

BRAISED COCO-NUTTY CABBAGE

1 tablespoon coconut oil

½ onion, finely chopped

½ head green savoy cabbage

½ cup (40 g) desiccated coconut

IN THE MORNING

1. Place the vegetables in the slow-cooker insert.

2. Season the beef with salt and pepper and place the beef on top of the vegetables. Add the rosemary and garlic then pour the stock over the beef.

3. For well-done beef, cover and cook for 8–10 hours on low or 4–5 hours on high. For medium beef, cook for 6–7 hours on low or 3–3½ hours on high.

IN THE EVENING

1. To make the Braised Coco-nutty Cabbage, heat the coconut oil in a saucepan and cook the onion until translucent. Toss through the cabbage and coconut then cook until the cabbage has wilted and coconut is golden. Serve the meat and vegetables straight from the slow cooker with the cabbage on the side.

Suggested Sides:
- Steamed courgettes
- Sweet Potato Mash (see page 132)

2. HEARTY IRISH BEEF STEW

This recipe isn't just for leftovers. Remember to double the cooking time if you're using uncooked meat.

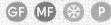

SERVES 4–6

PREPARATION TIME
15 minutes

COOKING TIME
4 hours on low
2 hours on high

3–4 portions leftover beef, shredded, or 500 g uncooked stewing beef

1 teaspoon sea salt

¼ teaspoon freshly ground black pepper

1 cup (115 g) sliced leek

1 onion, thinly sliced

4 stalks celery, roughly chopped

1 potato, peeled and cut into 3 cm cubes (you can use sweet potato if you prefer)

1 tomato, cut into quarters

1 teaspoon oregano

2 garlic cloves, chopped

½ cup (125 ml) stock of your choice

2 teaspoons sweet paprika

2–3 tablespoons arrowroot (if gluten-free or paleo) or cornflour, mixed to a paste in cold water

3 tablespoons flat-leaf parsley, finely chopped, to serve

1. Place all the ingredients into the slow-cooker insert. Cover and cook for 4 hours on low or 2 hours on high. Serve scattered with parsley.

Suggested Sides: • Thyme and Celeriac Mash (see page 132) or Gluten-free Damper (see page 30)

3. BEEF HASH

If you've got no leftover beef for this recipe you can use 400 g of beef mince instead.

SERVES 4–6

PREPARATION TIME
10 minutes

COOKING TIME
4 hours on low
2 hours on high

1 tablespoon olive oil

1 onion, finely chopped

1 garlic clove, crushed

⅓ cup (75 ml) Beginner's Beef Stock (see page 26) (or store-bought beef stock)

3–4 portions leftover beef, shredded (or whatever amount you have)

4 potatoes, washed and grated (skin on)

1 egg, whisked

2 fresh rosemary sprigs

2 teaspoons apple cider vinegar

sea salt and freshly ground black pepper, to taste

20 g butter

1. Combine all the ingredients except the leftover beef in the slow-cooker insert. Dot with the butter. Cover and cook for 4 hours on low or 2 hours on high. If you're using leftover beef add it to the slow cooker in the last 30 minutes of cooking to heat through.

2. Serve hot, once the potatoes have some colour.

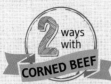

1. MEAL-IN-ONE CORNED BEEF WITH WHITE SAUCE

Use the leftover corned beef from this recipe to make the Reuben Deli Sandwich (see page 82).

(GF) (MF) ❄

SERVES 8–10

PREPARATION TIME
5 minutes

COOKING TIME
8 hours on low
4 hours on high

2 onions, quartered

1.3–1.5 kg corned beef silverside

4 cups (1 litre) Chicken Stock (see page 28) (or store-bought chicken stock)

4 tablespoons apple cider vinegar

freshly ground black pepper

2 bay leaves

4 cloves

3 carrots, roughly chopped

12 baby potatoes, halved

WHITE SAUCE

50 g butter

1 tablespoon gluten-free plain flour

4 tablespoons full-fat milk

⅓ cup (10 g) chopped flat-leaf parsley

IN THE MORNING

1. Place the onion in the slow-cooker insert. Rinse the corned beef thoroughly under cold water. Place in the slow cooker on top of the onion. Add the chicken stock, vinegar and enough water to cover the meat. Add the pepper, bay leaves and cloves. No need to season with salt – the corned beef will be salty enough. Cook for 8 hours on low or 4 hours on high.

IN THE EVENING

1. In the last 1–2 hours of cooking add the carrots and potatoes (tucked in around the sides and base of the beef).

BEFORE SERVING

1. Remove the meat and vegetables from the cooking liquid and cover to keep warm.

2. To make the white sauce, heat the butter in a small saucepan over low–medium heat. Stir in the flour. Remove from the heat. Gradually stir in 2 cups (500 ml) of the strained cooking liquid from the slow cooker. Return to heat and gradually add the milk. Continue stirring until the mixture boils and thickens. Stir through the parsley.

3. Slice the beef and serve with the vegetables and white sauce.

Suggested Sides: • Steamed greens or a garden salad

2. REUBEN DELI SANDWICH

*Ever wondered what to do with all that corned beef after a Sunday roast?
We've come up with a fresh take on a classic Reuben sandwich – Katz's Deli
style. Usually it's laden with sweet sauce and served on stodgy white bread
but this one will leave you feeling satisfied not stuffed.*

SERVES 6

PREPARATION TIME
5 minutes

COOKING TIME
3 hours on low
1½ hours on high

2 cups (300 g) leftover corned beef,
sliced or shredded (or deli-sliced salt
beef, if you like)

2 cups (450 g) homemade or store-
bought sauerkraut (made with salt or
whey only, not vinegar or sugar)

1 tablespoon caraway seeds

2 cups (225 g) grated Emmental cheese

12 slices rye sourdough

THOUSAND ISLAND DRESSING

1 cup (250 ml) whole egg mayonnaise

½ tablespoon rice malt syrup

½ teaspoon Dijon mustard

1 tablespoon harissa paste

juice of ½ lemon

sea salt and freshly ground
black pepper, to taste

1. Place the beef in the slow-cooker insert, sprinkle the sauerkraut on top
    and then the caraway seeds. Scatter the cheese on top. Cover and cook for
    3 hours on low or 1½ hours on high.

2. To make the Thousand Island Dressing, combine all the ingredients in a
    jar and shake until combined. Alternatively, whizz it up using a hand-held
    blender.

3. Serve the corned beef mixture between two slices of rye sourdough, topped
    with the dressing.

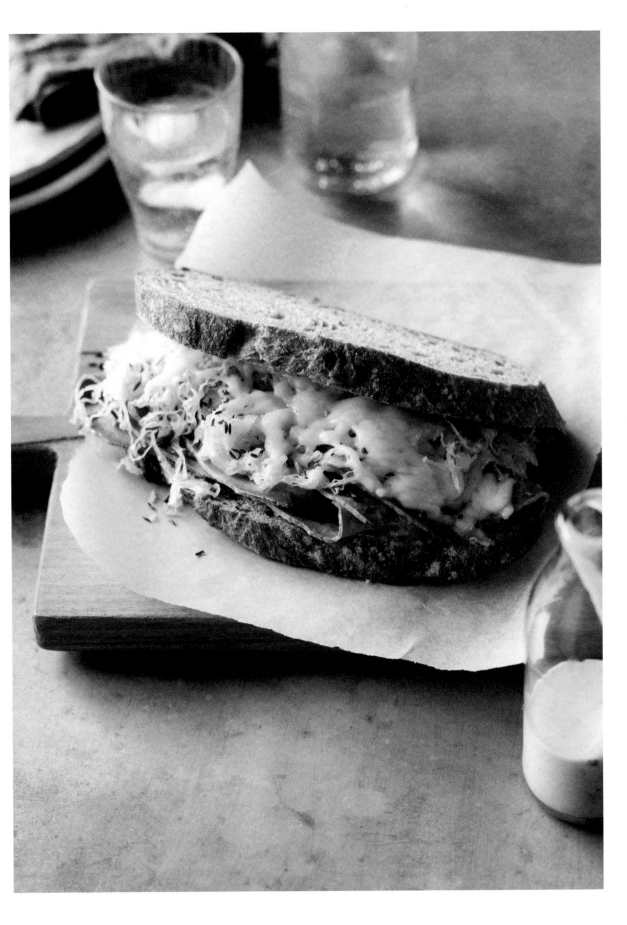

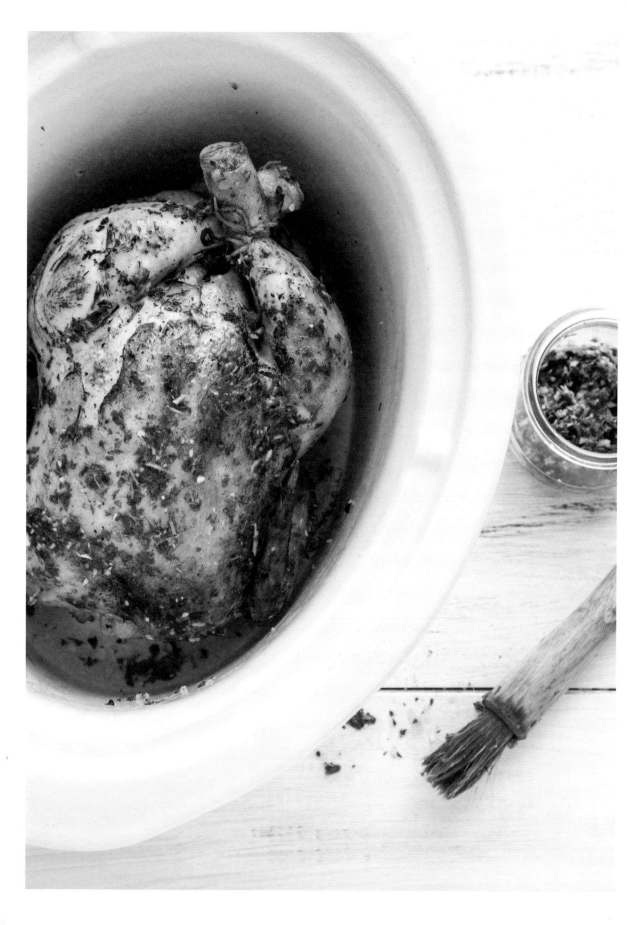

SARAH'S PICNIC CHICKEN WITH LEMONY GREMOLATA

GF MF ❄

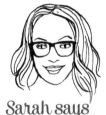

Sarah says

     " I slow-cooked a roast chicken for the office moonlight cinema picnic. I toted my slow cooker into the office, popped the pre-browned bird in with some herbs, turned it on and went about my day. So simple. Note: It's best to pre-brown the chicken for this recipe if you can. **"**

SERVES 6–8

PREPARATION TIME

5 minutes

COOKING TIME

6 hours on low
3 hours on high

1.5 kg whole organic chicken

2 lemons, unpeeled, roughly chopped

5 garlic cloves, unpeeled, smashed with the back of your knife

1 bunch rosemary

kitchen string (any string made of cotton or hemp)

100 g butter

⅔ cup (150 ml) white wine

1 cup (250 ml) Chicken Stock (see page 28) (or store-bought chicken stock, or water)

1 cup (250 ml) Lemony Gremolata (see page 67)

1. Wash the chicken and pat dry. Stuff the bird from the bottom end (where the legs are) with the lemon, garlic and rosemary. No need to be delicate. Tie the legs with kitchen string (cross the legs at the knuckle for a snugger fit).

2. Melt the butter in a hot frying pan and brown the chicken all over.

3. Place the chicken in the slow-cooker insert upside down (to keep the meat juicy).

4. Add the wine to the frying pan and bring to the boil. Pour the wine mixture over the chicken. Add the stock or water and cover with the lid. Cook for 6 hours on low or 3 hours on high.

5. Once cooked, remove the chicken and baste with the Lemony Gremolata before serving with your choice of sides.

TRICKY TIP

Freeze the leftover juices from the slow cooker in ice-cube trays to use as gelatinous and super-nutritious stock cubes in other recipes.

Suggested Sides: • Braised Coco-nutty Cabbage (see page 79), steamed greens or Easy Slaw (see page 97)

• Citrus-spiced Sweet Potatoes (see page 130)

MARGARET FULTON'S SCOTCH BROTH

SERVES 6–8

PREPARATION TIME
10 minutes

COOKING TIME
8–10 hours on low
4–5 hours on high

3 lamb shanks

½ cup (100 g) pearl barley, washed

1 onion, finely chopped

2 carrots, chopped

2 stalks celery, sliced

1 small swede, parsnip or turnip, chopped

6 cups (1.5 litres) Leftovers Vegetable Stock (see page 27) (or store-bought vegetable stock)

sea salt and freshly ground black pepper, to taste

fresh flat-leaf parsley, finely chopped, to serve

IN THE MORNING

1. Place the shanks in the slow-cooker insert along with the barley, vegetables and stock. Cover and cook for 8–10 hours on low or 4–5 hours on high.

IN THE EVENING

1. Remove the shanks from the slow cooker and pull away the meat from the bones. Roughly dice the meat, removing any fat or gristle. Skim any fat from the top of the soup, return the meat to the slow cooker and season to taste.

2. Serve very hot, sprinkled with the fresh parsley.

Suggested Sides:
- Steamed greens or tenderstem broccoli
- Sweet Potato Mash (see page 132)

KATE GIBBS' SLOW-COOKED PORK SHOULDER WITH BEER, KALE AND CRACKLING

❄

SERVES 6–8

PREPARATION TIME
15 minutes

COOKING TIME
6 hours on low
3 hours on high

2.5 kg deboned pork shoulder

sea salt

2 tablespoons fennel seeds

5 garlic cloves, peeled

zest of 1 lime

1 large bunch kale,
stalks removed

1 cup (250 ml) stout

juice of 3 limes

2 tablespoons rice malt syrup

1 tablespoon olive oil

2 teaspoons ground cinnamon

freshly ground black pepper,
to taste

lime wedges, to serve

1. Preheat the oven to 220°C/gas 7. If the pork is tied, remove the string. Use a razor or sharp knife to score the skin at 2 cm intervals, without cutting all the way to the meat (or ask your butcher to do this). Rub the skin with approximately ½ tablespoon salt. Use a sharp knife to carefully remove the skin from the pork in one piece. Place the pork skin, fat side down, on a shallow baking tray. Roast for 30–40 minutes, or until small bubbles form on the surface and the rind is golden and crisp. Remove from the oven and set aside.

2. Meanwhile, using a mortar and pestle, smash the fennel seeds, garlic and lime zest to make a paste. Rub the mixture all over the pork, getting it over all surfaces.

3. Place the kale leaves in the bottom of the slow-cooker insert, pushing them down a little. Place the pork on top.

4. Whisk together the remaining ingredients in a medium bowl and pour over the pork, adding salt and pepper to taste. Cover and cook for 6 hours on low or 3 hours on high until the pork is very tender.

5. Carve the pork and serve with kale, a drizzle of sauce from the slow cooker, shards of crackling, and lime wedges.

BEEF BRISKET 'N' BEER WITH GRAVY

SERVES 6

PREPARATION TIME
10 minutes

COOKING TIME
8–10 hours on low
4–5 hours on high

1.5–2 kg rolled beef brisket or silverside, trimmed of fat (for what to do with excess fat see page 17)

sea salt and freshly ground black pepper, to taste

2 onions, finely sliced

1 cup (250 ml) beer (a dark malty one is best)

1 tablespoon rice malt syrup

1 garlic clove, crushed

½ teaspoon dried thyme or 1 fresh sprig

1 bay leaf

3–4 carrots, peeled and halved lengthways

4 potatoes, washed and cut into chunks

2–3 tablespoons arrowroot or cornflour, mixed to a paste in cold water

IN THE MORNING

1. Rub the meat with salt and pepper. Place half the onion in the slow-cooker insert, then the meat and then the remaining onion. In a bowl combine the beer, rice malt syrup, garlic, thyme and bay leaf.

2. Pour the beer mixture over the meat and then tuck the veggies around the edges. Cover and cook for 8–10 hours on low or 4–5 hours on high.

BEFORE SERVING

1. Take the meat and veggies out of the slow cooker and cover to keep warm. Slowly pour the arrowroot or cornflour paste into the liquid in the slow cooker, stirring as you go. Cook on high with the lid off until the mixture thickens and reduces.

Suggested Sides:
- Cooked Quinoa (see page 42)
- Steamed greens or broccoli

WHEN HIPSTERS DISCOVERED THE SLOW COOKER

We noticed the daggy slow cooker has been making quite a comeback. Funky inner-city cafes and upscale restaurants are all using this handy kitchen appliance to revive their menus. This chapter has a few weird and kooky creations that would appeal to any hipster.

SPICED BACON JAM

Use this bacon jam like you would a relish. Have it on the side of a cheese board or indulge and serve it as a spread on a cheese toastie.

MAKES 1½ cups (375 ml)

PREPARATION TIME
5 minutes

COOKING TIME
5½ hours on low
3½ hours on high

400 g bacon, chopped finely (the finer the chop, the better the consistency)

1 large onion, finely chopped

3 garlic cloves

3 tablespoons rice malt syrup

1 teaspoon ground cinnamon

1 teaspoon ground ginger

1 tablespoon cider vinegar

1. Combine all the ingredients in the slow-cooker insert. Cover and cook for 5 hours on low or 3 hours on high, stirring halfway, until the bacon has softened.

2. Remove the lid and cook for a further 30 minutes on high until the mixture is syrupy and thick. Blitz the bacon jam in a food processor to desired consistency, or leave as is and store in an airtight container or sealed jar for up to 1 week in the fridge.

> **TRICKY TIP**
>
> This bacon jam is best served fresh, as the fat content will cause it to solidify in cool temperatures. Before serving, lightly reheat in the microwave or on the stovetop.

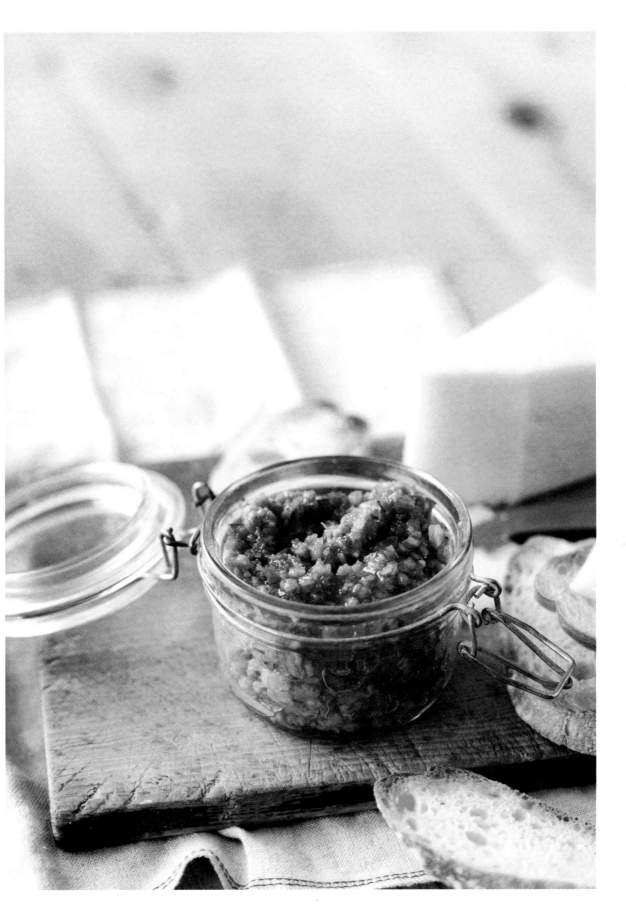

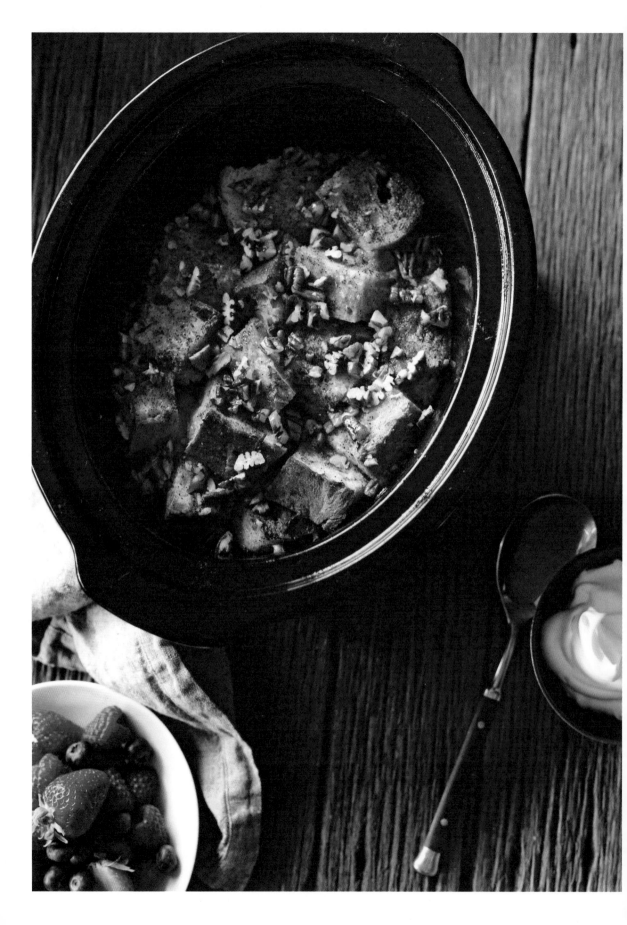

FRENCH TOAST PUDDING

This eggy pudding is packed with spices and topped with nuts. Simply yum!
Serve the pudding in the slow cooker at a dinner party for a bit of theatre.

SERVES 6–8

PREPARATION TIME
10 minutes
(+ overnight)

COOKING TIME
4 hours on low
2 hours on high

coconut oil or butter, for greasing

1 loaf bread, cut into 4 cm cubes
(any leftover bread will work for this)

6 eggs, whisked

2 cups (500 ml) milk (any type will
work fine)

4 tablespoons rice malt syrup

½ cup (125 ml) Pumpkin Purée (see
page 32)

1 tablespoon ground cinnamon

60 g butter, softened

½ cup (60 g) pecans, roughly chopped

2 teaspoons ground nutmeg

cream and fresh berries, to serve

THE NIGHT BEFORE

1. Grease the inside of the slow-cooker insert with the coconut oil or butter and
   add the cubes of bread. In a bowl, combine the eggs, milk, half the rice malt
   syrup, pumpkin and cinnamon and pour over the bread. Cover and let the
   bread mixture soak overnight in the fridge.

ON THE DAY

1. In a small bowl, combine the butter, remaining rice malt syrup, pecans
   and nutmeg.

2. Dollop on the top of the bread mix. Cover and cook for 4 hours on low
   or 2 hours on high. Serve warm with the cream and berries.

COFFEE AND CACAO-CURED BRISKET

The beauty of this brisket is the sensory overload you'll get from the moment you turn the slow cooker on. The smell of the smoky brisket will waft through the house and entice your taste buds and the spice rub will ensure that the meat stays moist and juicy. When serving, slice finely and make sure everyone gets a flavoursome chunk of the marinade!

SERVES 8–10

PREPARATION TIME
5 minutes
(+ 2 hours or overnight)

COOKING TIME
9 hours on low
5 hours on high

1.5–2 kg beef brisket

Easy Slaw (see page 97), to serve

pickles and homemade Tomato Sauce (see page 27), to serve

SPICE RUB

4 tablespoons rice malt syrup

3 tablespoons finely ground dark roast coffee

2 tablespoons raw cacao powder

1 tablespoon smoked paprika

2 teaspoons chilli powder

2 teaspoons sea salt

2 teaspoons garlic powder

2 teaspoons ground cumin

1. Place the brisket in the slow-cooker insert. Pour over the spice rub ingredients and massage into the brisket, ensuring the whole piece of meat is coated. Cover and refrigerate for at least 2 hours or overnight.

2. Cook brisket for 9 hours on low or 5 hours on high until the meat is tender. Serve with a side of Easy Slaw, pickles and homemade Tomato Sauce.

Suggested Sides: • Steamed green beans or Swiss chard

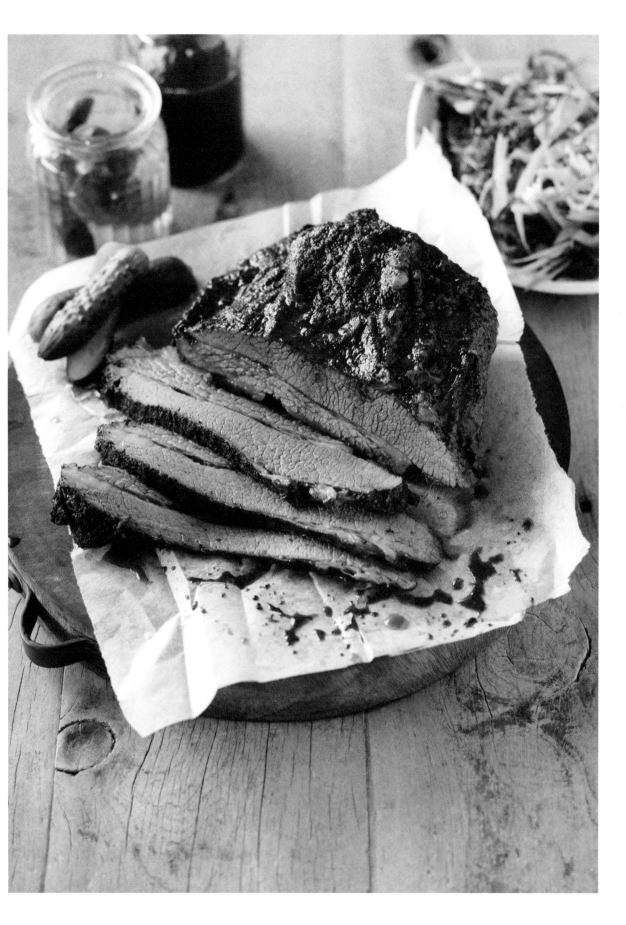

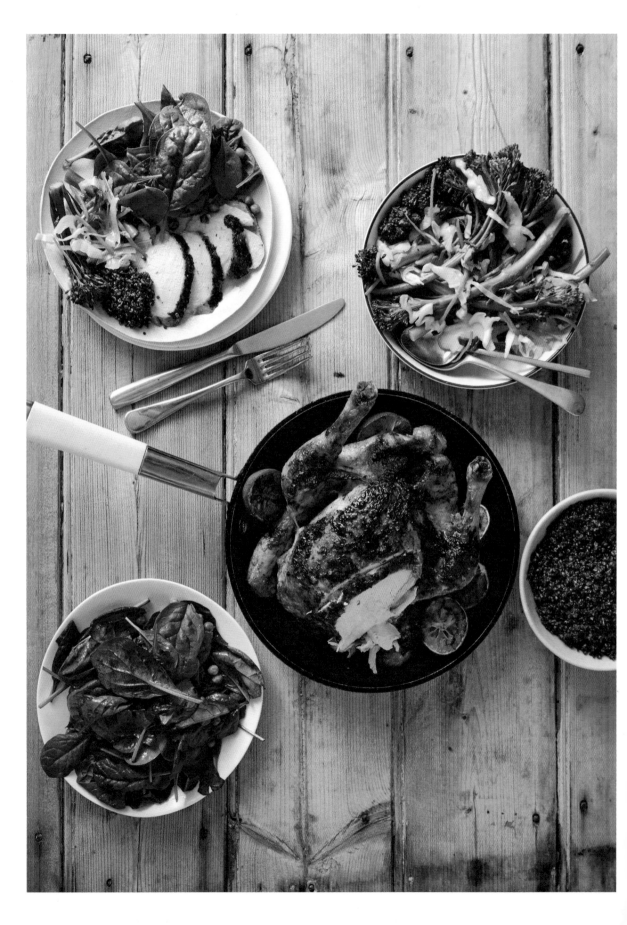

JUICY JERK CHICKEN
WITH EASY SLAW

SERVES 6

PREPARATION TIME
10 minutes

COOKING TIME
6 hours on low
3½ hours on high

40 g butter

1.5–1.8 kg whole organic chicken

juice of 3 limes

1 tablespoon ground allspice

1 teaspoon ground cinnamon

½ teaspoon cayenne pepper

2 teaspoons sea salt

1 tablespoon rice malt syrup

EASY SLAW

1 tablespoon olive oil

2 bunches tenderstem broccoli, halved lengthways

1 pack pre-shredded coleslaw mix

4 spring onions, sliced

IN THE MORNING

1. Melt the butter in a hot frying pan and brown the chicken all over. Remove from the pan and place it upside down in the slow-cooker insert.

2. Combine the lime juice with the spices and salt in the same pan over low heat. Add the rice malt syrup and stir until melted and combined.

3. Pour the mixture over the upside-down chicken and rub all over, including the cavity, to coat thoroughly.

4. Cover and cook for 6 hours on low or 3½ hours on high.

IN THE EVENING

1. To make the Easy Slaw, heat the olive oil in a large saucepan, then gently sweat the broccoli until almost tender. Add the remaining ingredients and stir until warmed through.

2. Remove the chicken from the slow cooker and slice the meat from the bone. Serve with slaw.

Suggested Sides: • Cooked Quinoa (see page 42) or
Citrus-spiced Sweet Potatoes (see page 130)

PEANUT BUTTER GRANOLA

MAKES 5 cups
(about 500g)

PREPARATION TIME
10 minutes

COOKING TIME
4 hours on low
2 hours on high

1½ tablespoons coconut oil or butter

⅓ cup (75 g) peanut butter (smooth or crunchy)

4 tablespoons rice malt syrup (optional)

3 cups (180 g) coconut flakes

2 cups (250 g) unsalted mixed nuts, roughly chopped

2 tablespoons chia seeds

1 teaspoon ground cinnamon (optional)

pinch of sea salt

full-fat natural yoghurt or coconut cream, to serve

1. Stir the coconut oil, peanut butter and rice malt syrup in a small pan over low heat, or in the microwave, until combined. Place the coconut flakes, nuts, chia seeds, cinnamon and salt in the slow-cooker insert. Pour over the peanut butter mixture and stir to combine.

2. Cover and cook for 4 hours on low or 2 hours on high, stirring occasionally. Turn off the slow cooker and remove the lid for 30 minutes to allow the granola to cool down and dry out. Store in a sealed container for up to 2 weeks. Serve with yoghurt or coconut cream.

KOREAN KIMCHI AND BEEF

GF

SERVES 6

PREPARATION TIME
10 minutes

COOKING TIME
8 hours on low
4 hours on high

1 kg chuck steak, cut into chunks

1 cup (225 g) kimchi (store-bought or homemade)

SAUCE

3 garlic cloves, crushed

2 teaspoons chilli powder

freshly ground black pepper, to taste

3 tablespoons rice wine

3 tablespoons tamari or soy sauce

4 tablespoons water

2 teaspoons rice malt syrup

1. Combine the sauce ingredients in the slow-cooker insert.

2. Place the beef in the slow-cooker insert and cover with the sauce. Stir to combine.

3. Cover and cook for 8 hours on low or 4 hours on high. Stir through the kimchi and serve with your choice of sides.

Suggested Sides:
- Steamed Asian greens
- Cooked Quinoa (see page 42)

A LITTLE OFFALY CHAPTER

For some, offal is a sensitive topic, which is why we're starting slow. Try these easy recipes and you might just have a new appreciation for nose-to-tail eating!

ALL DAY, EVERY DAY PÂTÉ

MAKES 3 cups (about 1 kg)

PREPARATION TIME
10 minutes

COOKING TIME
6 hours on low
3 hours on high

60 g butter

1 onion, chopped

1½ cups (150 g) roughly chopped mushrooms

3 garlic cloves, crushed

½ teaspoon sea salt

½ teaspoon freshly ground black pepper, to taste

1 teaspoon ground nutmeg

1 kg ox liver, cut into 5 cm pieces

½ cup (125 ml) cream

½ cup (15 g) chopped flat-leaf parsley

1. Heat the butter in a large frying pan over medium heat. Add the onion, mushrooms, garlic, salt, pepper and nutmeg. Sauté for 5 minutes, stirring frequently until softened.

2. Add the liver to the pan and stir well for 30 seconds, until the liver is browned.

3. Pour the mixture into the slow-cooker insert. Cover and cook for 6 hours on low or 3 hours on high.

4. Transfer the mixture to a shallow dish and allow to cool for 15 minutes.

5. Place in a blender or food processor and add the cream. Blend until smooth. Stir in the parsley.

6. Scoop the pâté into a serving dish and refrigerate for 1 hour before serving. This pâté will last 1–2 days in a sealed container in the fridge.

Suggested Sides:
- Sourdough or crackers
- Olives and cheese

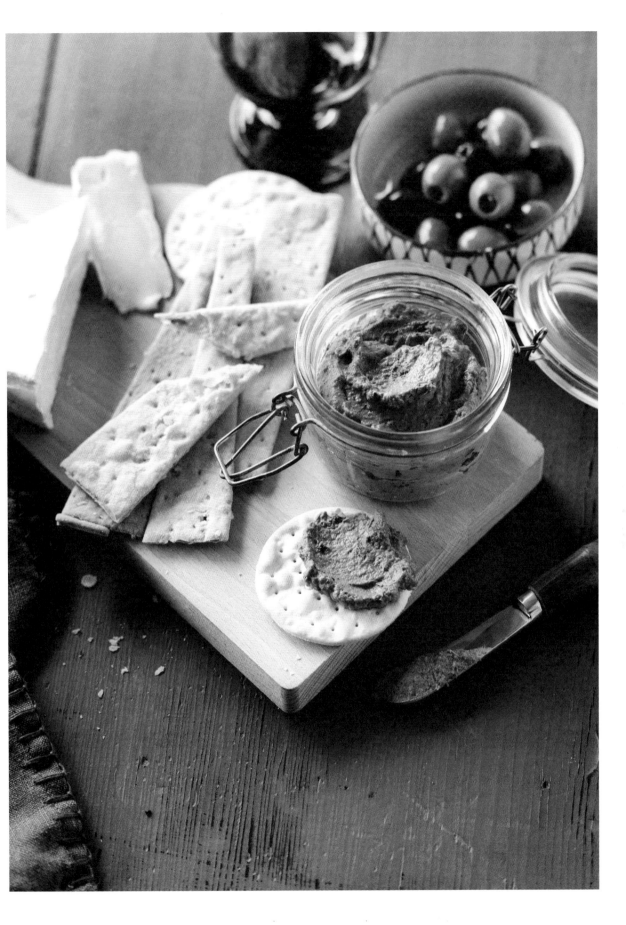

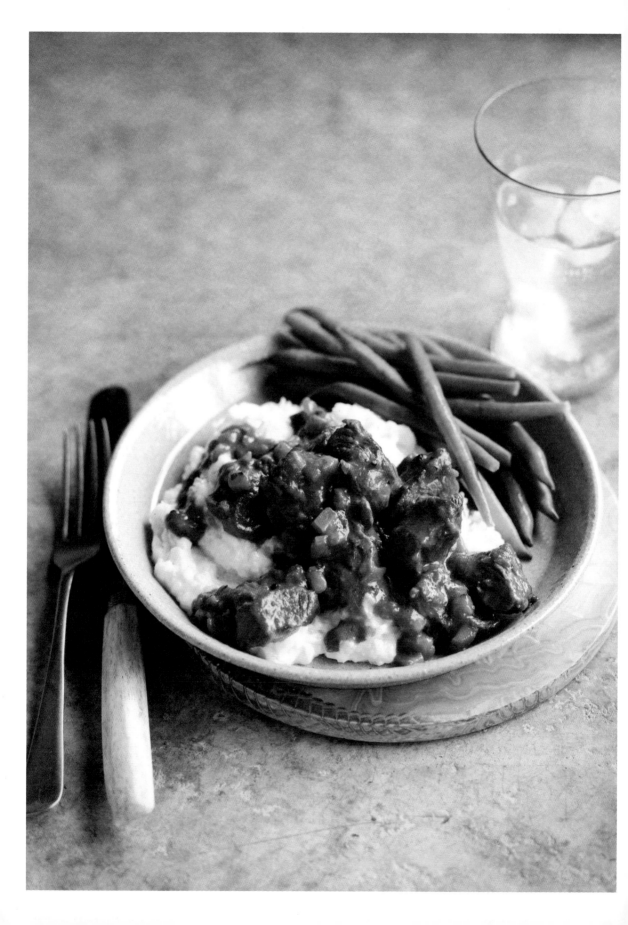

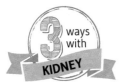

ways with
KIDNEY

1. MUM'S STEAK AND KIDNEY STEW

GF MF ❄

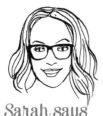

Sarah says

" Mum's original recipe came from a little cookbook that her local butcher gave her when she first got married at 21. It espoused eating cheap cuts and eating a little meat at each meal, including breakfast (with carbs and sugar very much limited). These principles were very much pivotal in my early eating. This dish was always made on Dad's birthday. He claims it's his favourite meal, but I think much of the delight was derived from watching my brothers' discomfort at eating offal. "

SERVES 6

PREPARATION TIME

15 minutes

COOKING TIME

10 hours on low
5 hours on high

1 onion, sliced

2 carrots, finely chopped

1½ cups (150 g) sliced mushrooms

2 garlic cloves, sliced

2 tablespoons gluten-free plain flour

¼ teaspoon sea salt

½ teaspoon freshly ground black pepper

½ teaspoon dried mixed herbs (or dried rosemary)

1 kg stewing beef (chuck is best, or blade), cubed

2–4 lamb kidneys (or 1 ox kidney), cored (remove the gristle on the inside with a small knife) and cut into small pieces

¾ cup (175 ml) Beginner's Beef Stock (see page 26) (or store-bought stock)

1. Place the onion, carrot, mushrooms and garlic in the slow-cooker insert. In a bowl, combine the flour, salt, pepper and herbs together and coat the meat and kidneys. Add the meat and dry mixture to the insert. Pour over the stock, cover and cook for 10 hours on low or 5 hours on high.

TRICKY TIP

Reserve leftover portions to use in the Steak and Kidney Cheat's Pie or the Steak and Kidney Stew with Herby Dumplings (see page 104).

Suggested Sides: • Sweet Potato Mash (see page 132), Cauliflower Cream (see page 111) or steamed greens

2. STEAK AND KIDNEY CHEAT'S PIE

SERVES 4–6

PREPARATION TIME
5 minutes

COOKING TIME
10 hours on low
5 hours on high

2 sheets puff pastry

20 g butter, melted

Mum's Steak and Kidney Stew
(see page 103)

1. Preheat the oven to 190°C/gas 5. Remove the puff pastry from the freezer about 10 minutes before serving. Cut each pastry sheet into six squares. Place on a lined baking tray, brush with melted butter and bake in the oven for 6–8 minutes until golden and puffy.

2. Serve the stew in small bowls or ramekins with two pastry puffs on top.

3. STEAK AND KIDNEY STEW WITH HERBY DUMPLINGS

SERVES 4–6

PREPARATION TIME
5 minutes

20 g butter, chopped

1½ cups (175 g) gluten-free self-raising flour

½ teaspoon sea salt

2 teaspoons chopped thyme

2 teaspoons chopped flat-leaf parsley

2–3 tablespoons full-fat milk

1 quantity Mum's Steak and Kidney Stew (see page 103)

TO MAKE THE HERBY DUMPLINGS

1. In a bowl, rub the butter into the flour and salt with your fingertips until the mixture resembles fine breadcrumbs. Add the herbs and mix to a soft dough with the milk. Using about 2 tablespoons of mixture, roll into small balls.

TO COOK DUMPLINGS

1. Thirty minutes before the end of cooking time, remove the lid from the slow cooker and place the dumplings on top of the stew. Lay greaseproof paper over the slow-cooker insert and cover with the lid. Cook for 30 minutes on high until the dumplings are cooked.

> ### TRICKY TIP
>
> Prepare these dumplings in advance and freeze them uncooked. When you plan to use them, remove from the freezer to thaw and cook as per instructions.

STUFFED LAMBS' HEARTS

Our general manager, Zoe, licked her lips at the thought of sharing her nan's best offaly dish. Give it a go. We promise you'll be gobsmacked by how downright delish it is! You'll need kitchen string for this recipe.

SERVES 6

PREPARATION TIME
15 minutes

COOKING TIME
6 hours on low
3 hours on high

6 organic lamb hearts

12 rashers bacon

1 litre Beginner's Beef Stock (see page 26) or Chicken Stock (see page 28) (or store-bought stock)

2 bay leaves

1 teaspoon arrowroot (if gluten-free or paleo) or cornflour, mixed to a paste in cold water

STUFFING

20 g butter

2 red onions, finely chopped

1 cup (100 g) finely chopped mushrooms

4 garlic cloves, crushed

1½ cups (370 ml) red wine

1 cup (50 g) breadcrumbs or 1 cup (185 g) Cooked Quinoa (see page 42) (for gluten-free or paleo version)

sea salt and freshly ground black pepper, to taste

1 tablespoon finely chopped sage leaves

1 teaspoon dried rosemary

TO MAKE THE STUFFING

1. In a saucepan, melt the butter and cook the onion, mushroom and garlic until soft. Add the wine and allow the liquid to reduce by half. Add the breadcrumbs or Cooked Quinoa. Season with salt and pepper and add the sage and rosemary. Set aside to cool.

TO PREP THE HEARTS

1. Trim the hearts of any excess fat and sinew (especially around the opening). Remove any clots from the ventricles using a spoon or your finger (your butcher can also do this for you). Using your fingers, fill the hearts with the stuffing.

2. Place a rasher of bacon over the opening of each heart to prevent stuffing falling out and wrap around. Place another rasher crossways and secure the bacon around each heart with string.

3. Stand the hearts next to each other in the slow-cooker insert. Add the stock and bay leaves. Cover and cook for 6 hours on low or 3 hours on high. Remove the hearts and set aside to keep warm.

4. Pour the remaining sauce into a saucepan and reduce on the stove until slightly thickened. If you want to thicken the sauce further, stir in the arrowroot paste or cornflour and stir vigorously over low heat until thickened. Serve the hearts with gravy and your choice of sides.

Suggested Sides: • Thyme and Celeriac Mash (see page 132)

• Steamed courgettes and green beans, or other greens

SWEETBREAD BURRITOS

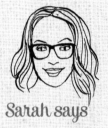

Sarah says

" This was a bit of an experimental dish (that worked beautifully!) to combine really cheap beef and some offal (for maximum nutrition and to make it as appealing as possible). I made it for my mates Rick and Brad and they barely flinched when I told them they were eating lamb's thalamus. When you buy sweetbreads, have a chat to your butcher about what variety you're getting. In some countries, sweetbreads are, in fact, calf pancreas or thalamus glands (to be honest it doesn't really matter which you wind up with). It's often advised to soak sweetbreads in cold water for a few hours first, changing the water several times to remove impurities. I found this really wasn't necessary for this recipe. My butcher agrees. Check with yours. "

SERVES 6

PREPARATION TIME
15 minutes

COOKING TIME
8 hours on low
4 hours on high

2 onions, finely chopped

1 green pepper, chopped

4 garlic cloves, crushed

1 bunch coriander, stalks finely chopped (reserve leaves for serving)

1 kg beef brisket, diced

400 g sweetbreads, cut into 1.5 cm cubes

2 tablespoons tomato purée

1½ teaspoons ground cumin

1 teaspoon cayenne pepper

1 teaspoon dried oregano

¾ cup (175 ml) Beginner's Beef Stock (see page 26) (or store-bought beef stock)

6 burrito wraps, warmed

1. Place the onion, green pepper, garlic and coriander stalks in the slow-cooker insert. Place the meat and sweetbreads on top, dollop over the tomato purée, herbs and spices and then pour the stock over the lot.

2. Cover and cook for 8 hours on low or 4 hours on high. Spoon the mixture onto the burrito wraps and top with your choice of sides.

Suggested Sides:
- Fresh coriander leaves
- Lime wedges
- Easy Slaw (see page 97)
- Sliced avocado
- Sour cream, yoghurt or grated cheese

SAME-SAME BUT DIFFERENT

We've given your favourite sauce-laden recipes an IQS makeover.

CHINESE BEEF CHEEKS

This dish is super rich and loaded with flavour. Serve it with rice or quinoa and plenty of steamed green veggies to balance things out.

SERVES 6

PREPARATION TIME
10 minutes
(+ overnight)

COOKING TIME
7 hours on low
3½ hours on high

5–6 beef cheeks (approx. 1.5 kg), fat trimmed (it can be quite thick) and each cheek cut into 2–3 even-sized pieces

1 bunch spring onions, finely chopped

4 cm knob ginger, grated

5 garlic cloves, finely sliced

1 bird's eye chilli, finely sliced

1 teaspoon Chinese five-spice powder

1 teaspoon granulated stevia (optional)

⅓ cup (75 ml) Chinese rice wine

4 tablespoons soy sauce or tamari (preferably low salt)

2 cups (200 g) sliced mushrooms (shiitake or brown)

1 cup (250 ml) Beginner's Beef Stock (see page 26) (or store-bought beef stock)

½ cup (125 ml) water

1 extra spring onion, finely sliced

THE NIGHT BEFORE

1. Combine all the ingredients except the mushrooms, stock, water and extra spring onion in the slow-cooker insert. Cover and refrigerate overnight.

IN THE MORNING

1. Place the mushrooms on top and pour over the stock and water. Cook for 7 hours on low or 3½ hours on high. Serve sprinkled with the extra sliced spring onion.

Suggested Sides:
- Steamed Asian greens (pak choi works well) or steamed broccoli
- Cooked Quinoa (see page 42) or jasmine rice

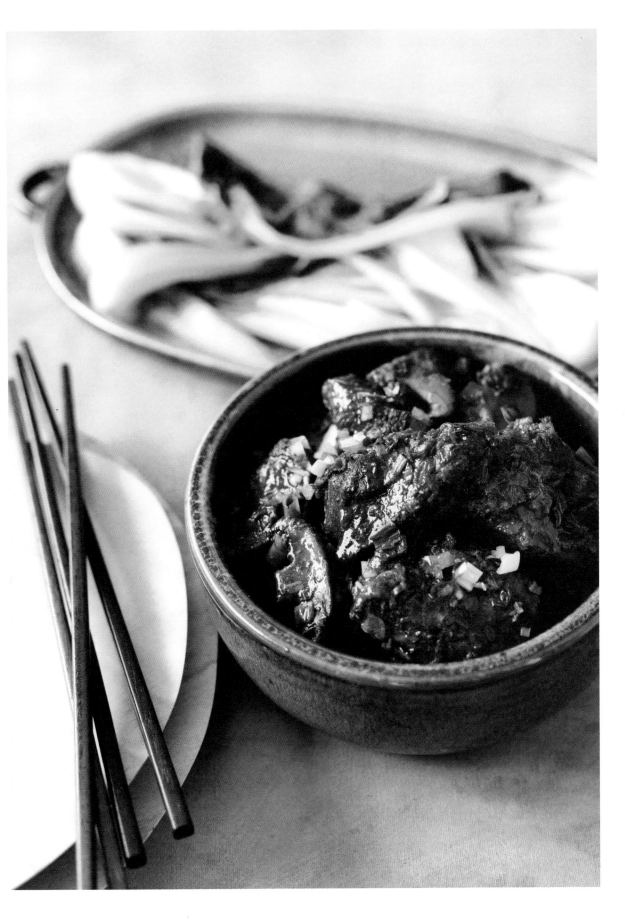

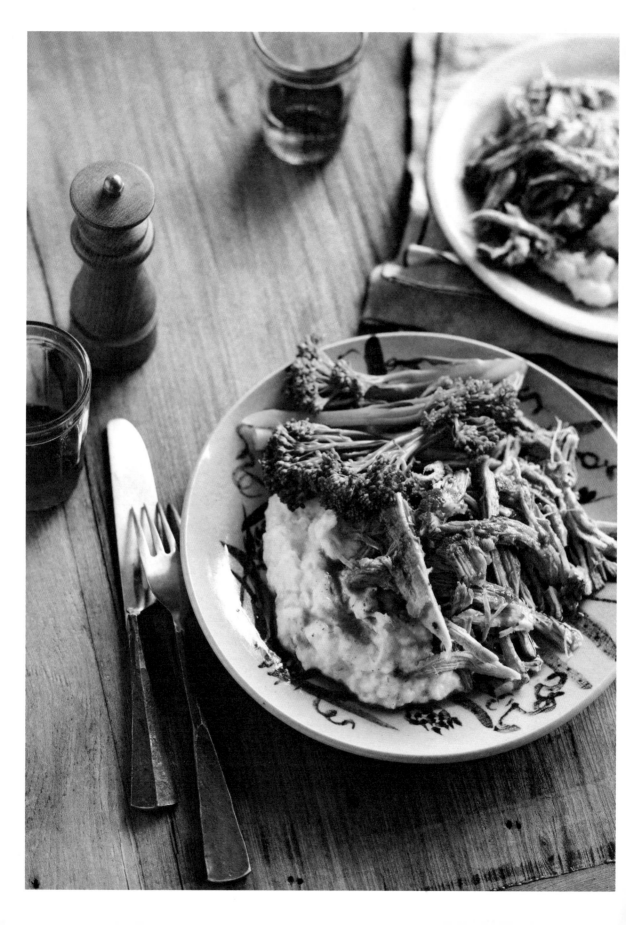

'BARBECUED' PULLED PORK WITH CAULIFLOWER CREAM

This recipe has all the sweetness and smokiness of a traditional barbecued pulled pork without the sickly sweet sauce.

SERVES 6–8

PREPARATION TIME
10 minutes
(+ 2 hours or overnight)

COOKING TIME
8 hours on low
4 hours on high

2 teaspoons fennel seeds

1½ teaspoons whole black peppercorns

1 tablespoon sea salt

1 tablespoon smoked paprika

1 teaspoon ground cumin

1 teaspoon ground allspice (or ground cinnamon)

2 teaspoons ground chilli (or chilli flakes)

1–1.5 kg piece of pork shoulder (preferably bone in), or pork neck

2 tomatoes, chopped into quarters

2 garlic cloves, crushed

2 bay leaves

½ cup (125 ml) red wine or stock (any type is fine)

⅓ cup (75 ml) cider vinegar

CAULIFLOWER CREAM

½ head cauliflower, broken into small florets

⅔ cup (150 ml) cream

20 g butter

sea salt and freshly ground black pepper, to taste

THE NIGHT BEFORE

1. Finely grind the fennel and peppercorns with a mortar and pestle or spice grinder. Add the salt and remaining spices and mix to combine.

2. Rub the spice blend over the meat, rubbing well into the fatty bits, massaging it all over. Place the coated meat in the slow-cooker insert, cover and refrigerate for at least 2 hours (or overnight, for a stronger flavour).

IN THE MORNING

1. Place the insert in the slow cooker and add the remaining ingredients. Cook for 8 hours on low or 4 hours on high.

BEFORE SERVING

1. When the pork has 20 minutes to go, place the cauliflower, cream and butter in a saucepan and cook, covered, over a low heat for 15–20 minutes or until soft. Season to taste and purée until smooth.

2. Transfer the pork to a plate and use two forks to shred the meat apart. Put the shredded meat back in the slow cooker for another 20 minutes with the sauce. Cook on high, uncovered, until warmed through.

Suggested Sides:
- Cooked Quinoa (see page 42)
- Steamed greens (tenderstem broccoli works well)

PORK AND FETA MEATBALLS

The sweet veggies in this dish will collapse to form the sauce for your courgette 'pasta'. Allow them to cook down in the slow cooker until you're happy with the softness. Bon appétit!

SERVES 6

PREPARATION TIME
10 minutes

COOKING TIME
5 hours on low
2½ hours on high

4 stalks celery, finely chopped

2 carrots, finely chopped

1 large fennel bulb, thinly sliced

750 g pork mince

1 small onion, finely grated

2 garlic cloves, crushed

¼ cup (25 g) almond meal

2 eggs, lightly whisked

½ cup (60 g) crumbled feta

2 teaspoons fennel seeds

4 tablespoons flat-leaf parsley, finely chopped

½ cup (125 ml) Chicken Stock (see page 28) (or store-bought chicken stock)

½ x 400 g can chopped tomatoes

6 cups (900 g) courgette noodles/ ribbons or grated courgettes

grated parmesan, to serve

1. Place the celery, carrots and fennel in the slow-cooker insert.

2. In a large bowl, combine the pork, onion, garlic, ground almonds, eggs, feta, fennel seeds and parsley, using your hands for best results. Roll tablespoons of the mixture into balls. Place the balls on top of the vegetables in the slow cooker (it's okay if you have to stack a few on top of each other).

3. Combine the stock and tomatoes and pour over the meatballs. Cover and cook for 5 hours on low or 2½ hours on high.

4. Serve the meatballs with the courgettes and veggies. Pour the remaining sauce from the slow cooker over the top and scatter with the parmesan. We like to lightly pan-fry our courgettes in coconut oil before serving. This enhances the flavour and helps your body digest the courgettes.

> **TRICKY TIP**
>
> If the sauce is still quite runny, remove the lid and cook on high for 30 minutes until it thickens.

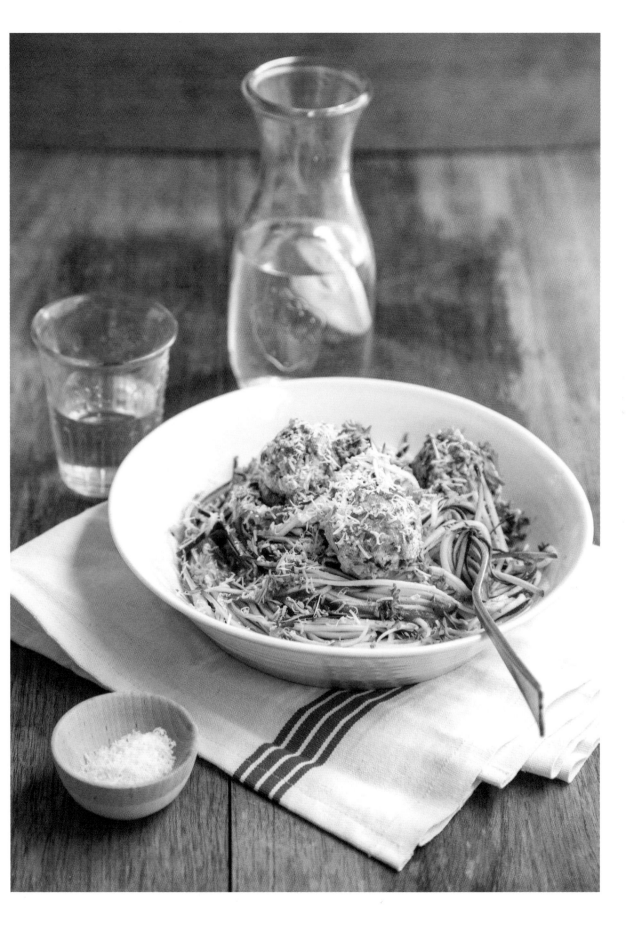

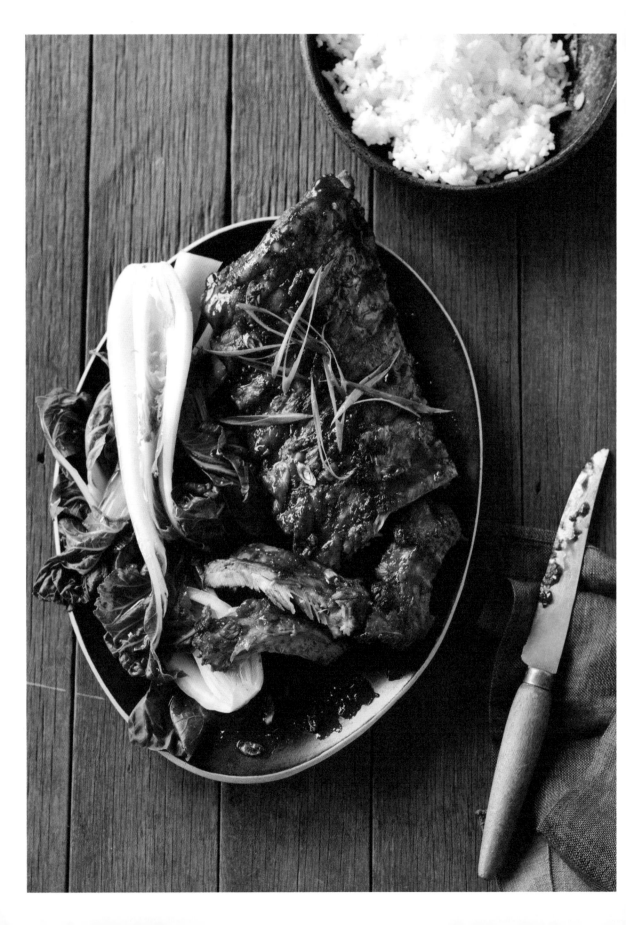

CHAR SIU PORK RIBS

These ribs are finger-licking good! As they cook they become super tender and the meat falls off the bone. Enjoy with some steamed greens and drizzle the excess sauce over a bed of jasmine rice.

SERVES 6

PREPARATION TIME
10 minutes
(+ overnight)

COOKING TIME
8 hours on low
4 hours on high

2 tablespoons olive oil

1.5 kg pork ribs (or chicken wings for a cheaper alternative)

1 cup (250 ml) Chicken Stock (see page 28) (or store-bought chicken stock)

3 spring onions, thinly sliced (save the green ends as a garnish)

CHAR SIU SAUCE

½ cup (125 ml) tamari

2 tablespoons smooth peanut butter

⅓ cup (75 ml) rice malt syrup

4 tablespoons Chinese shaosing or rice wine

2 teaspoons cider vinegar

1 teaspoon Chinese five-spice powder

2 teaspoons sesame oil

2 teaspoons grated fresh ginger

2 garlic cloves, crushed

1 long red chilli, finely chopped

THE NIGHT BEFORE

1. Heat the oil in a large frying pan and brown the pork ribs.

2. In a small bowl, prepare the Char Siu Sauce by whisking all the ingredients together.

3. Place the ribs in the slow-cooker insert and pour the Char Siu Sauce over the meat. Toss to combine. Cover and place in the fridge overnight to marinate.

IN THE MORNING

1. Place the slow-cooker insert into the cooker. Pour over the stock and scatter the spring onions on top. Cover and cook for 8 hours on low or 4 hours on high.

BEFORE SERVING

1. When the ribs are tender, remove them from the slow cooker, wrap in aluminium foil and place in a low oven to stay warm. Turn the slow cooker up to high and reduce the sauce, with the lid off, for 15–20 minutes until sticky (or desired consistency). Garnish with spring onion ends.

Suggested Sides:
- Steamed Asian greens
- Jasmine rice or Cooked Quinoa (see page 42)

ROO ROGAN JOSH
WITH A CUCUMBER RAITA

This is a great way to eat sustainable, healthy meat. Don't be put off by the use of kangaroo in this recipe. The curry sauce masks any 'gamey' flavour.

SERVES 6

PREPARATION TIME
10 minutes

COOKING TIME
6 hours on low
3 hours on high

800 g kangaroo steak, diced
(or beef chuck steak, if you prefer)

2 teaspoons ground coriander

2 teaspoons ground cardamom

2 teaspoons ground cumin

2 teaspoons smoked paprika

½ teaspoon cayenne pepper

2 onions, finely sliced

4 cm knob ginger, grated

4 garlic cloves, crushed

½ cup (125 ml) Beginner's Beef Stock
(see page 26) (or store-bought
beef stock)

½ x 400 g can chopped tomatoes

2 bay leaves

1 long red chilli, finely chopped

1 x 400 ml can coconut milk

fresh coriander leaves, to serve

CUCUMBER RAITA

1 cup (250 ml) Probiotic Greek Yoghurt
(see page 31) (or natural full-fat
yoghurt)

1 ridge cucumber, deseeded
and finely chopped

2 tablespoons mint leaves

sea salt and freshly ground black
pepper, to taste

squeeze of lemon juice (optional)

1. Place the steak in the slow-cooker insert. Add the spices, onion, ginger, garlic, stock, tomatoes, bay leaves, chilli and coconut milk. Stir to combine. Cover and cook for 6 hours on low or 3 hours on high until the meat is tender.

2. While the curry is cooking, make the Cucumber Raita by combining all the ingredients in a small bowl. Serve the curry scattered with the coriander leaves, with Raita and your choice of sides.

Suggested Sides: • Basmati rice or Cooked Quinoa (see page 42)

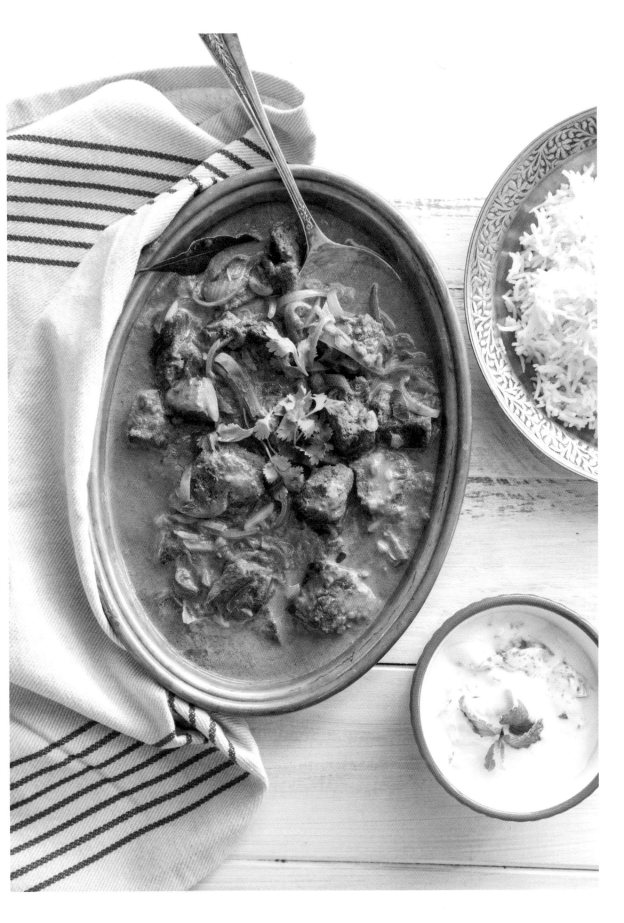

RETRO
SLOPPY JOES

This is a fun meal to dish out on football Grand Final day when everyone is sitting around focused on the TV.

SERVES 6

PREPARATION TIME
5 minutes

COOKING TIME
8 hours on low
4 hours on high

1 kg turkey or beef mince

1 green or red pepper, finely chopped

1 onion, finely chopped

½ x 400 g can chopped tomatoes

4 tablespoons Dijon or English mustard

4 tablespoons apple cider vinegar

2 tablespoons rice malt syrup

3 garlic cloves, crushed

1 teaspoon ground cinnamon

1 teaspoon cayenne pepper

sea salt and freshly ground pepper, to taste

8 bread rolls, split horizontally

8 slices tasty cheese (optional)

1. Place the mince in the slow-cooker insert. Add all the remaining ingredients, except the rolls and cheese. Stir until the mince is coated. Cover and cook for 8 hours on low or 4 hours on high.

2. Once cooked, stir again. Using a ladle, scoop the mixture into the rolls. Top with cheese, if you like. Serve straight away.

TRICKY TIP

Keep any leftovers for a protein-packed breakfast the following day.

Suggested Sides:
- Fresh baby spinach
- Thinly sliced cucumber

PIZZA PEPPERS

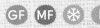

SERVES 6

PREPARATION TIME
5 minutes

COOKING TIME
8 hours on low
4 hours on high

6 red or yellow peppers

600 g beef or turkey mince

1 onion, finely chopped

1 garlic clove, crushed

1 cup (185 g) Cooked Quinoa
(see page 42)

2 teaspoons tamari or soy sauce

1 teaspoon paprika

¼ teaspoon dried sage

2 tablespoons tomato purée

1 teaspoon sea salt

1 cup (115 g) grated cheddar

½ cup (125 ml) warm water

1. Cut the tops off the peppers and use in a salad or throw into another
   slow-cooker meal. Remove the seeds and membrane.

2. In a bowl, combine the mince, onion, garlic, Cooked Quinoa, tamari, paprika,
   sage, tomato purée and salt. Mix well. Fill the peppers with the mixture.

3. Place the peppers upright in the slow-cooker insert. Top with the cheddar.
   Pour the warm water around the base of the peppers.

4. Cover and cook for 8 hours on low or 4 hours on high until the meat
   is fully cooked through and the cheese has melted.

Suggested Sides: •   Steamed greens (mangetout, beans or tenderstem
broccoli work well)

'THE VIETNAMESE CHICKEN CURRY THAT MADE SARAH CRY'

GF ❄ P

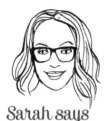

Sarah says

❝ Okay, so when I'm asked to cite my favourite food experience, this is the one I share. I first ate *cari ga* on a mountain-bike trip with my brother Pete in Vietnam. We'd been riding for nine hours through a desert and one of the highest mountains in the country, plus I had food poisoning. By the time I arrived, I was dead-set delirious and my brother found us the closest hole-in-the-wall place, steaming from a cauldron of this Vietnamese version of chicken curry. At the first spoonful, I cried. Then I ordered two more serves. ❞

SERVES 6

PREPARATION TIME
10 minutes
(+ overnight)

COOKING TIME
8 hours on low
4 hours on high

700 g chicken thighs or pieces, with skin on and bone in

1 stalk lemongrass, peeled and thinly sliced (only use the cream end, reserve the green end)

2 garlic cloves, crushed

3 cm knob ginger, grated (or 1 tablespoon store-bought grated ginger)

2 tablespoons fish sauce

½ cup (125 ml) yellow curry paste or Massaman curry paste

1 cup (250 ml) Chicken Stock (see page 28) (or store-bought chicken stock)

2 sweet potatoes, roughy chopped

1 large carrot, roughly chopped

1 x 400 ml can coconut milk

½ teaspoon granulated stevia

2 bay leaves

2–3 tablespoons arrowroot (if gluten-free or paleo) or cornflour, mixed to a paste in cold water

2 spring onions, finely sliced

roti, mountain bread or poppadoms to serve

THE NIGHT BEFORE

1. Place the chicken, lemongrass, garlic, ginger, fish sauce and half the curry paste in the slow-cooker insert. Toss to combine. Cover and refrigerate for at least an hour or, in this case, overnight.

IN THE MORNING

1. Place the insert into the slow cooker and add in the remaining curry paste, stock, vegetables, coconut milk, stevia, leftover lemongrass and bay leaves. Stir to combine. Cook for 8 hours on low or 4 hours on high.

IN THE EVENING

1. If you like a thicker curry, 20 minutes before serving stir in the arrowroot or cornflour paste. Cook on high with the lid off for 20 minutes until the sauce thickens.

2. Garnish with the spring onions and serve with roti, mountain bread or poppadoms.

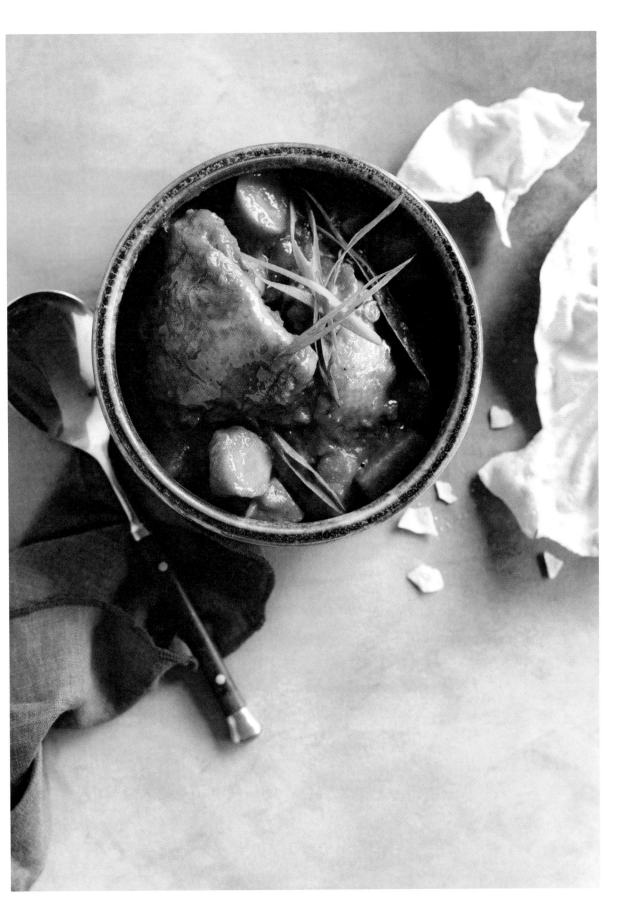

'MAPLE SYRUP' PORK BELLY WITH PECANS

Pork belly is a very fatty, rich piece of meat, but beautifully succulent. Be sure to eat it with plenty of greenery.

SERVES 6

PREPARATION TIME
15 minutes

COOKING TIME
7 hours on low
3½ hours on high

1 kg piece pork belly, cut into 6 thick slices

⅓ cup (75 ml) rice malt syrup

2 cinnamon sticks

1 long red chilli, finely chopped

8 whole cloves

3 garlic cloves, crushed

⅓ cup (75 ml) tamari or soy sauce

½ cup (125 ml) Chicken Stock (see page 28) (or store-bought chicken stock)

½ orange, rind grated and flesh deseeded and cut into segments

3 tablespoons apple cider vinegar

½ cup (60 g) pecans, preferably activated and toasted lightly in a pan

IN THE MORNING

1. Place the pork slices in the slow-cooker insert, fatty-side up (try to wedge them all so that they fit in one layer). Pour over the syrup then add the remaining ingredients. Cover and cook for 7 hours on low or 3½ hours on high.

BEFORE SERVING

2. Remove the pork and cover to keep warm. Skim as much of the fat from the top of the liquid as you can, reserving it in a jar. (For what to do with leftover fat see page 17).

3. Strain the liquid through a fine sieve into a large jug, removing the cinnamon and other whole spices, then return to the slow-cooker insert. Cook on high with the lid off, about 20 minutes. Serve the pork and sauce with your choice of sides.

> **TRICKY TIP**
>
> If the top of your pork hasn't browned in the slow cooker, place on a foil-lined baking tray and place under a hot grill for 5 minutes to crisp up, while you thicken the liquid.

Suggested Sides:
- Sweet Potato Mash (see page 132)
- Steamed tenderstem broccoli and sautéed kale

A FEW CLEVER SIDES

Make some simple sides in your slow cooker to go with your favourite dish. If you have two slow cookers, you can make a main and side dish at the same time. Not a bad idea if you entertain a lot!

CIDER-GLAZED BEETS

Running out of room in the oven? Chuck these beets in the slow cooker.
Seriously, they taste like they've been oven-roasted.

SERVES 6

PREPARATION TIME
5 minutes

COOKING TIME
6 hours on low
3 hours on high

2 bunches beetroot (or 12 beetroots), scrubbed and cut into halves

1 tablespoon rice malt syrup, melted

2 tablespoons water

2 tablespoons cider vinegar

1 teaspoon dried mixed herbs

1 garlic clove, crushed

1. Place the beetroot, rice malt syrup, water, vinegar, herbs and garlic in the slow-cooker insert. Stir until the beetroot is combined with the seasoning.

2. Cover and cook for 6 hours on low or 3 hours on high. The beetroot should give when pricked with a knife.

3. Serve with the juices from the pan poured over the top of the beetroot.

MEDITERRANEAN RATATOUILLE

SERVES 6–8

PREPARATION TIME
10 minutes

COOKING TIME
6 hours on low
3 hours on high

1 tablespoon olive oil

1 large aubergine, cut into 4 cm cubes

300 g pumpkin or squash, peeled and cut into chunks

1 red pepper, thinly sliced

1 red onion, finely diced

2 courgettes, cut into small chunks

1 x 400 g can chickpeas, rinsed and drained

2 garlic cloves, crushed

2 teaspoons dried basil

1 teaspoon dried oregano

½ x 400 g can chopped tomatoes

100 g feta

fresh rosemary or basil, to serve

1. Place all the ingredients, except the feta and rosemary or basil, in the slow-cooker insert. Toss to combine.

2. Cover and cook for 6 hours on low or 3 hours on high until the vegetables are softened and cooked through.

3. Serve with the feta crumbled over the dish, scattered with rosemary or basil.

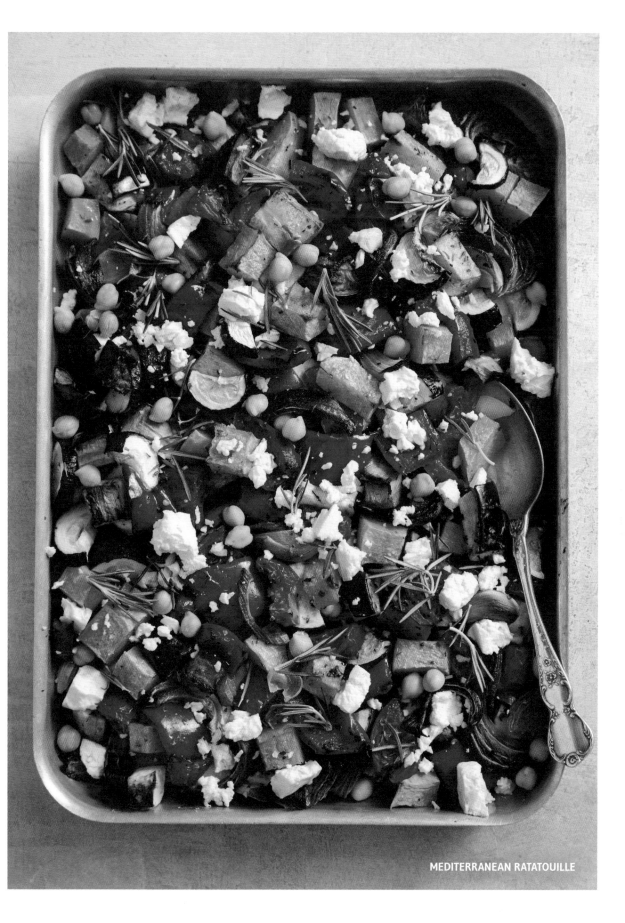

MEDITERRANEAN RATATOUILLE

MAC AND CAULI-CHEESE

This classic cheesy dish has a few sneaky ingredients to transform it into a proper meal. Make it for the kids or your partner and see if they notice the difference.

SERVES 6

PREPARATION TIME
5 minutes

COOKING TIME
3 hours on low
1½ hours on high

coconut oil or butter, for greasing

2 cups (600 g) cauliflower florets, broken into bite-sized pieces or blitzed in a blender

2 cups (225 g) macaroni (gluten-free, if you prefer)

3 cups (350 g) grated cheddar

½ teaspoon paprika (optional)

½ teaspoon mustard powder (optional)

2 cups (500 ml) full-fat milk

sea salt and freshly ground black pepper, to taste

1. Grease the inside of the slow-cooker insert with the coconut oil or butter.

2. Add the cauliflower, macaroni, 2 cups (225 g) of the cheese, paprika, mustard and milk. Season and stir to combine. Sprinkle the remaining cheese on top.

3. Cover and cook for 3 hours on low or 1–2 hours on high. If there's any excess oil from the cheese, skim off or pat with kitchen paper. Remove the lid and cook uncovered for a further 15–20 minutes on high until the dish looks melted and creamy.

> **TRICKY TIP**
>
> Add in some peas when combining all the ingredients. They add a nice sweetness and a hit of greenery in a seriously cheesy dish!

'HONEY' MUSTARD ROOT VEGGIES

This is a great side to cook up for a dinner party when you're using the oven for other things. Simply throw in all the ingredients and turn it on!

SERVES 6–8

PREPARATION TIME
5 minutes

COOKING TIME
5 hours on low
2½ hours on high

coconut oil or butter, for greasing

5 carrots, peeled and roughly chopped

4 parsnips, peeled and roughly chopped

2 red onions, cut into wedges

1 large sweet potato, peeled and roughly chopped

4 tablespoons rice malt syrup

1 tablespoon English mustard

1 tablespoon olive oil

1 tablespoon fresh thyme, chopped (or 2 teaspoons dried thyme)

1 teaspoon sea salt and freshly ground black pepper

cider vinegar, to serve

1. Lightly grease the inside of the slow-cooker insert to avoid the veggies sticking. Place the carrot, parsnip and onion in the slow cooker. Top with the sweet potato.

2. In a bowl, mix the rice malt syrup, mustard, oil, thyme and salt and pepper until well combined. Pour over the vegetables and toss to ensure they are all coated. Cover and cook for 5 hours on low or 2½ hours on high until the vegetables are tender but not mushy. Drizzle a splash of cider vinegar over the vegetables before serving.

Variation: Thyme and Rosemary Root Veggies: To make this fragrant variation, complete step 1 and then combine 2 tablespoons olive oil with 4 fresh rosemary sprigs (or 2 teaspoons dried), 1 fresh thyme sprig (or 1 teaspoon dried), 1 sage sprig (or ½ teaspoon dried). Cover and cook for 5 hours on low or 2½ hours on high.

PEA AND SPINACH-Y DAHL

This is another great side to make for a dinner party when you're using the oven for other things. Simply throw in all the ingredients and press play.

SERVES 6

PREPARATION TIME
5 minutes

COOKING TIME
10 hours on low
5 hours on high

2 cups (400 g) dried yellow split peas

50 g butter or ghee

2 onions, finely chopped

2 garlic cloves, crushed

3 cm knob ginger, grated

1 long red or green chilli, finely chopped

1 teaspoon cumin seeds

1 teaspoon mustard powder

1 teaspoon ground coriander

1 teaspoon ground turmeric

1 teaspoon garam masala

½ x 400 g can chopped tomatoes

3 cups (750 ml) Leftovers Vegetable Stock (see page 27) (or store-bought stock)

2 cups (500 ml) water

½ teaspoon granulated stevia (optional)

2 cups (100 g) baby spinach, Swiss chard or kale, deveined and roughly chopped

fresh coriander leaves, to serve

IN THE MORNING

1. Rinse the peas under cold water until the water runs clear and drain well.

2. In a large frying pan, melt the butter or ghee. Add the onion, garlic, ginger and chilli. Cook until the onion is translucent.

3. Add the remaining spices and cook until the mixture is fragrant. Combine the mixture in the slow-cooker insert with the tinned tomato, stock, water, stevia and split peas.

4. Cover and cook for 10 hours on low or 5 hours on high.

IN THE EVENING

1. Stir the chopped greens through the warm dahl mixture until wilted. Serve with a scattering of coriander on top.

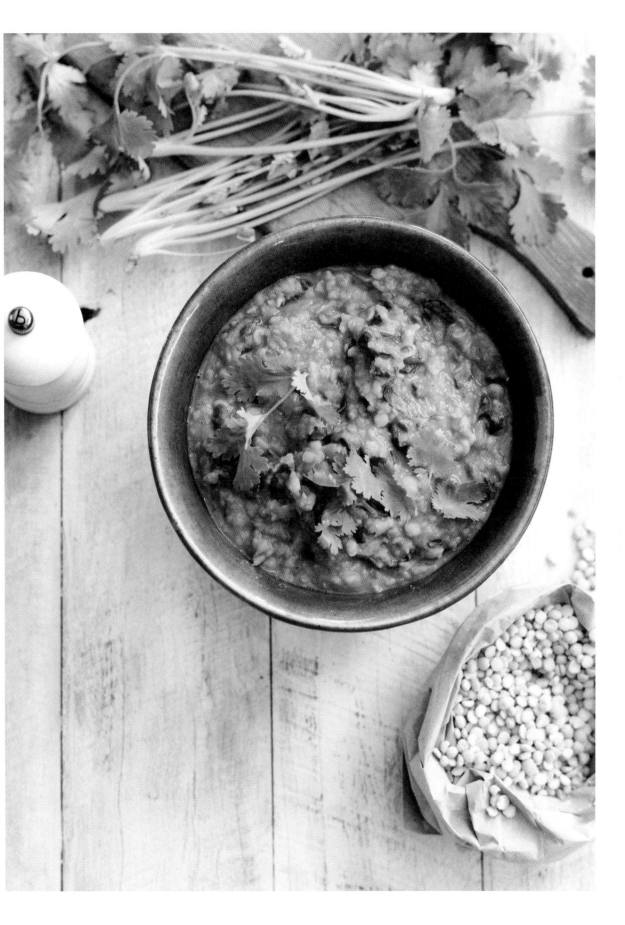

'CANDIED' SWEET POTATO CASSEROLE

Serve this as a dessert or for breakfast, if you like, with a dollop of full-fat natural yoghurt or cream.

SERVES 8

PREPARATION TIME
5 minutes

COOKING TIME
7 hours on low
3½ hours on high

coconut oil or butter, for greasing

4–5 sweet potatoes,
peeled and thickly sliced

½ cup (125 ml) rice malt syrup

2 teaspoons ground cinnamon

2 teaspoons vanilla powder

¼ teaspoon sea salt

½ cup (125 ml) unsweetened almond milk

½ cup (60 g) pecan halves, crushed

1 cup (250 ml) full-fat natural yoghurt or cream

1. Grease the inside of the slow-cooker insert. Layer in the sweet potato slices.

2. In a bowl, combine the rice malt syrup, cinnamon, vanilla powder, salt and almond milk. Pour the mixture evenly over the top of the sweet potatoes.

3. Sprinkle with the crushed pecans. Cover and cook for 7 hours on low or 3½ hours on high until soft. Mash with the back of a fork to the desired consistency. Serve with a dollop of natural yoghurt or cream.

CITRUS-SPICED SWEET POTATOES

These citrussy, sweet spuds are ideal for cutting through the richness of a slow-cooked meal.

SERVES 4–6

PREPARATION TIME
5 minutes

COOKING TIME
7 hours on low
3½ hours on high

4 large sweet potatoes, washed well and patted dry

1½ teaspoons sea salt

1½ teaspoons ground cumin

1½ teaspoons chilli powder or flakes

2 teaspoons olive oil

juice of 2 limes

¾ cup (175 ml) sour cream

1 bunch chives, finely chopped

1. Prick the sweet potatoes with a fork, 4–5 times per potato.

2. In a bowl, combine the salt and spices with the oil. Rub the spice mixture over the sweet potatoes to coat evenly.

3. Place the sweet potatoes in the slow-cooker insert, standing them vertically if you need to. Cover and cook for 7 hours on low or 3½ hours on high until soft when pierced with a knife.

4. Serve the sweet potatoes sliced down the centre. Squeeze over the lime juice, dollop with sour cream and sprinkle with chives.

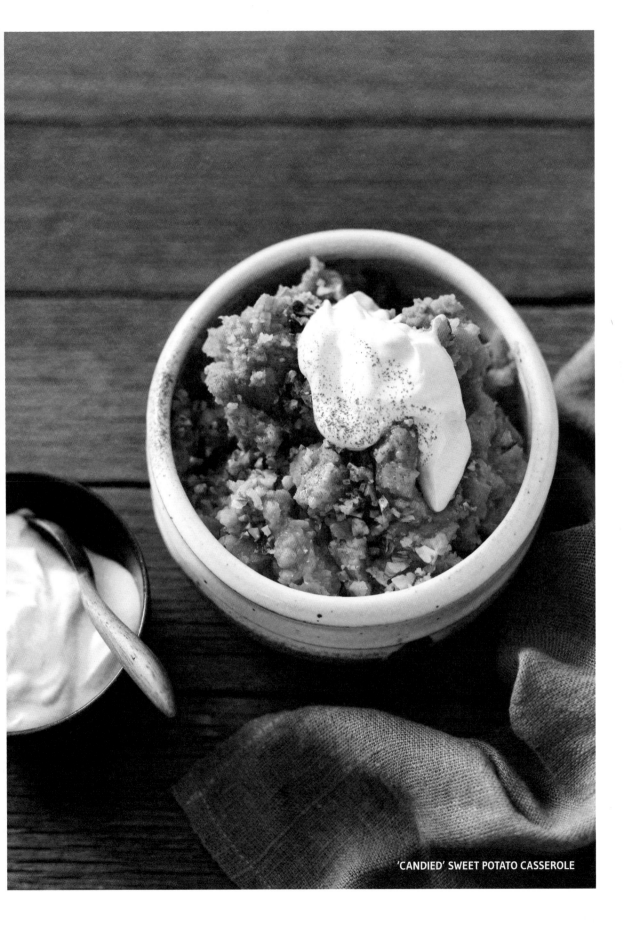

'CANDIED' SWEET POTATO CASSEROLE

SWEET POTATO MASH

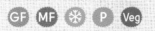

SERVES 6

PREPARATION TIME
5 minutes

COOKING TIME
6 hours on low
3 hours on high

800 g sweet potatoes, peeled, chopped into even chunks

60 g butter, diced

4 tablespoons full-fat milk or cream

sea salt and freshly ground black pepper, to taste

chives, finely chopped, to serve (optional)

1. Place the sweet potato in the slow-cooker insert. Cover and cook for 6 hours on low or 3 hours on high. It should be soft when pierced with a knife.

2. Add the butter and milk and season to taste. Using a stick blender or masher, mash until smooth. Serve sprinkled with chives if you like.

THYME AND CELERIAC MASH

SERVES 6

PREPARATION TIME
5 minutes

COOKING TIME
6 hours on low
3 hours on high

400 g potatoes, peeled and quartered

1 kg celeriac bulb, trimmed, peeled and roughly chopped

40 g butter, diced (or 4 tablespoons cream)

2–3 teaspoons Dijon mustard

2 teaspoons fresh thyme

¾ cup (175 ml) full-fat milk

sea salt and freshly ground black pepper, to taste

1. Place the potato and celeriac in the slow-cooker insert. Cover and cook for 6 hours on low or 3 hours on high until the potatoes are soft when pierced with a knife.

2. Add the butter, mustard, thyme, milk, salt and pepper to the potatoes. Using a stick blender or masher, mash to desired consistency. Serve.

> **TRICKY TIP**
>
> If you don't have a vegetable that's listed in the recipe, that's fine! Feel free to mix up the recipe with your favourite veggie combo.

CAKES AND PUDS

Yes, it's true – you can make moist, flavoursome cakes and puds in a slow cooker. Enjoy them for dessert or as a treat at morning tea.

CREAMY VANILLA RICE PUDDING

This recipe takes us back to Sunday dinners with the grandparents.
We've IQS-ified the traditional dessert so you can enjoy it without the sugar
dump (the usual recipe has up to 2 cups/450 g of the white stuff).

SERVES 12

PREPARATION TIME
5 minutes

COOKING TIME
6 hours on low
3 hours on high

1 cup (200 g) medium-grain white rice, uncooked

2 cups (500 ml) full-fat coconut cream

1 litre full-fat milk

⅓ cup (75 ml) rice malt syrup

5 cm piece orange rind

2 vanilla pods, halved with the seeds scraped out or 2 teaspoons vanilla powder

1 teaspoon ground cinnamon, plus extra to serve

pistachios and finely grated orange zest, to serve

1. Combine the rice, coconut cream, milk, rice malt syrup, orange rind, vanilla pod and seeds or powder and cinnamon in the slow-cooker insert. Stir well.

2. Cover and cook for 6 hours on low or 3 hours on high. Stir once or twice towards the end of the cooking time. The rice is cooked when it's tender and soft. Remove and discard the vanilla pods and orange rind. Serve sprinkled with pistachios, orange zest and cinnamon.

> **TRICKY TIP**
>
> For the first few hours, this recipe will look like nothing is happening. Don't worry, as soon as the rice starts to absorb the liquid it will thicken quite quickly. Keep an eye on it to avoid it burning and becoming gluggy. Serve immediately for the best texture.

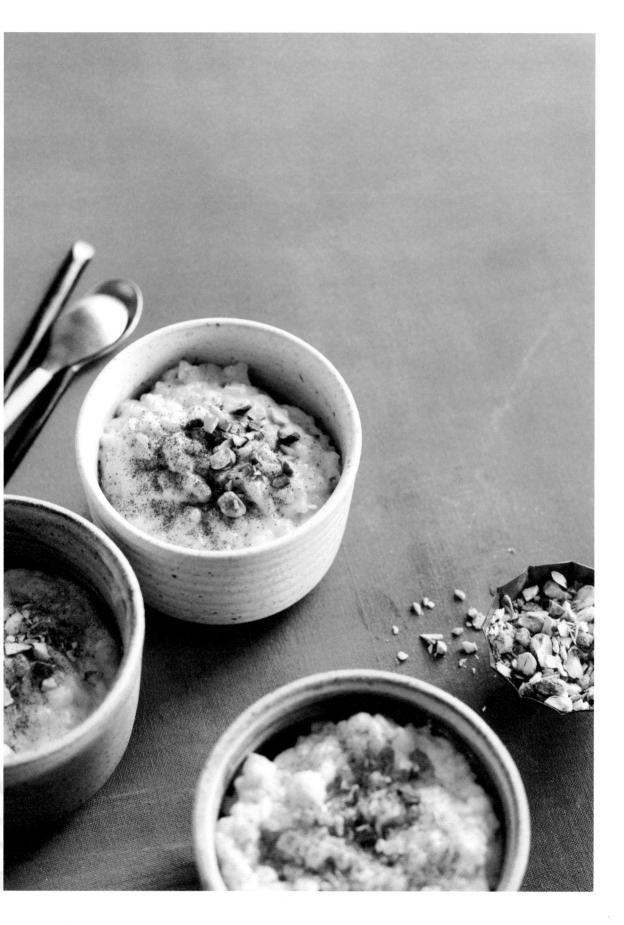

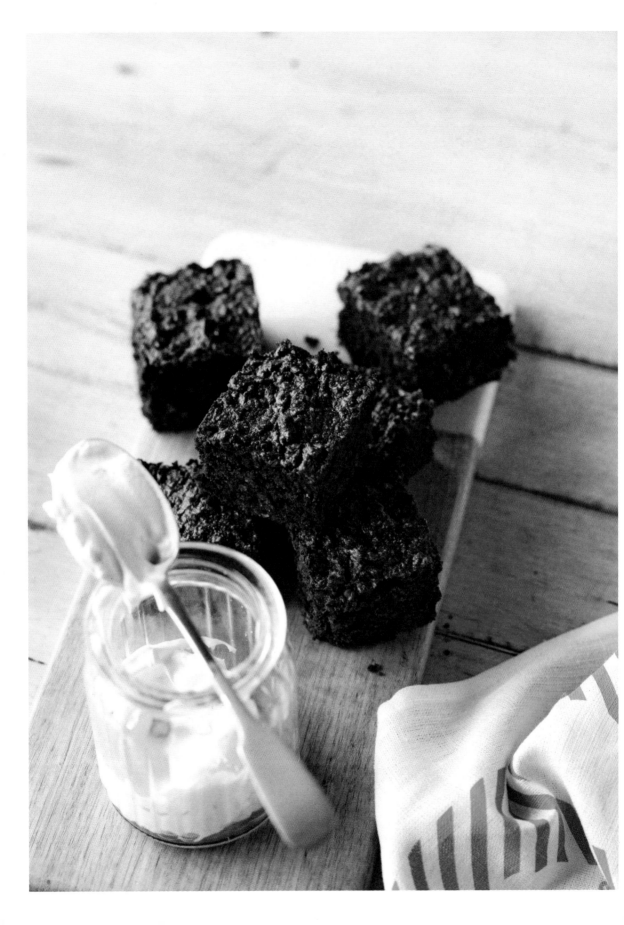

SLOW BRO'S (DOUBLE-CHOC WALNUT BROWNIES)

These brownies are a hit in the IQS office. You'll find the centre of the batch is moist and gooey and the sides have a nice chocolaty crust. Serve with some cream for ultimate indulgence.

SERVES 16

PREPARATION TIME
10 minutes

COOKING TIME
3 hours on low
2 hours on high

oil or butter, for greasing

1½ cups (150 g) ground almonds

½ cup (50 g) raw cacao powder

1 teaspoon gluten-free baking powder

½ teaspoon sea salt

125 g butter, melted (or ½ cup (100 g) melted coconut oil)

⅓ cup (75 ml) rice malt syrup

3 eggs

½ cup (60 g) walnuts, finely chopped

80 g dark (85% cocoa) chocolate, chopped into chunks

cream, to serve

1. Grease the inside of the slow-cooker insert and line with baking paper so that it reaches halfway up the sides.

2. In a large bowl, combine the ground almonds, raw cacao, baking powder and salt.

3. In a separate bowl, whisk the butter and rice malt syrup until well combined. Add the eggs and continue to whisk until the mixture comes together.

4. Pour the butter mixture into the dry ingredients and mix thoroughly. Stir through the walnuts and chocolate chunks.

5. Pour the batter into the prepared slow cooker. Cover and cook for 2½ hours on low or 1½ hours on high, until the exterior of the mixture is firm and the centre is no longer liquid. Remove the lid and continue cooking on low for a further 30 minutes or until the centre cooks through. The centre will always be more moist than the perimeter of the brownie; don't burn the outside waiting for the centre to firm up.

6. Switch off the slow cooker and leave the brownies to rest for 10–15 minutes. Carefully remove from the slow cooker by grabbing the edges of the baking paper and gently lifting out. Allow to cool completely before slicing. Serve with cream.

Variation: Peanut Butter Fudge Brownies: To make this delicious variation, omit the walnuts and, instead, stir through 4 heaped tablespoons of softened, crunchy, natural peanut butter in Step 4. Pour the mixture into prepared slow cooker. Cover and cook for 3 hours on low or 2 hours on high.

LIME, COCONUT AND POPPY SEED CAKE WITH ZESTY COCONUT BUTTER

This cake is so moist and light. Perfect with a cup of tea, which is how we like to enjoy it.

SERVES 12

PREPARATION TIME
10 minutes

COOKING TIME
3½ hours on low
2 hours on high

1½ cups (150 g) ground almonds

1 cup (125 g) gluten-free self-raising flour

1 teaspoon gluten-free baking powder

½ teaspoon sea salt

125 g unsalted butter, softened

½ cup (125 ml) rice malt syrup

2 eggs

juice and zest of 1 lime

1 teaspoon poppy seeds

ZESTY COCONUT BUTTER

2 cups (150 g) desiccated coconut

juice and zest of ½ lime

1. Grease the inside of the slow-cooker insert and line with baking paper so that it reaches halfway up the sides.

2. In a medium bowl, combine the ground almonds, flour, baking powder and salt. Set aside.

3. In a separate bowl, place the butter and rice malt syrup. Beat using an electric beater until combined and smooth. Beat in the eggs one at a time until creamy. Add the lime juice and zest and beat on low until smooth. Add the flour mixture and continue to beat until smooth. Fold through the poppy seeds.

4. Pour the cake batter into the prepared slow cooker. Cover and cook for 3½ hours on low or 2 hours on high until a skewer inserted into the centre comes out clean. The edges of the cake should be browned and starting to pull away from the sides.

5. Meanwhile, to make the Zesty Coconut Butter, blend the coconut until it forms a spreadable mixture. This can take up to 10 minutes depending on your blender. Stir through the lime juice. Add some zest if you like it extra citrussy.

6. Allow the cake to cool for 20 minutes in the slow cooker and then gently remove the cake by lifting up the sides of the baking paper.

7. Cut cake into slices and serve warm with Zesty Coconut Butter, if you like.

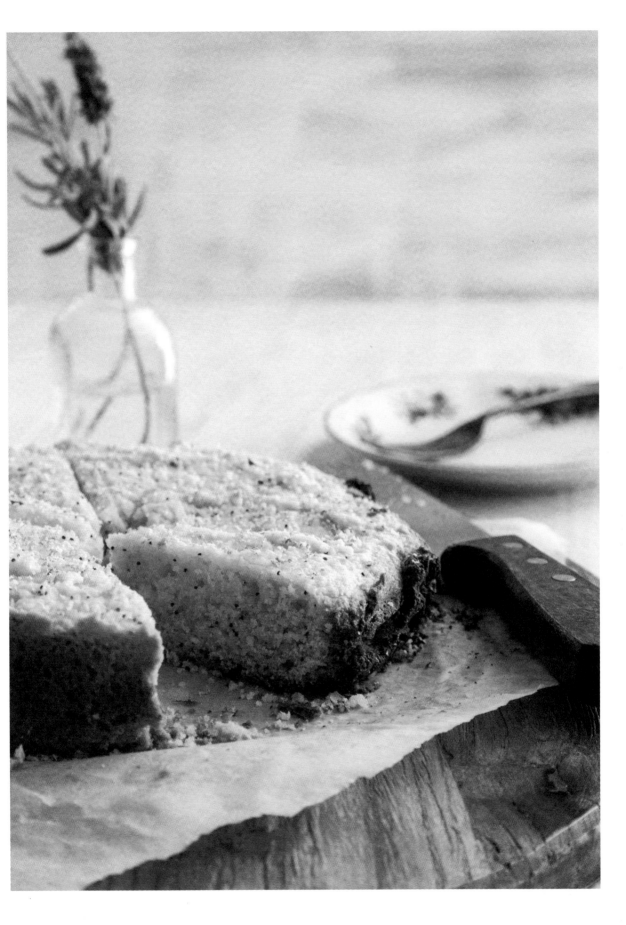

MIXED BERRY CLAFOUTIS

This recipe is best made in a 4.5 litre slow cooker. If yours is bigger you'll need to increase the quantities to suit.

SERVES 6

PREPARATION TIME
5 minutes

COOKING TIME
5½ hours on low
3 hours on high

oil or butter, for greasing

300 g frozen mixed berries

3 eggs

1 teaspoon vanilla powder

⅓ cup (75 ml) rice malt syrup

½ cup (125 ml) full-fat milk

½ cup (60 g) gluten-free self-raising flour

½ teaspoon orange zest

40 g butter, melted

½ cup (125 ml) coconut cream or pouring cream, to serve

1. Grease the inside of the slow-cooker insert and line with baking paper so that it reaches halfway up the sides.

2. Scatter the berries over the base evenly. Whisk together the eggs, vanilla powder and rice malt syrup until combined and fluffy. Add the milk, flour, orange zest and butter and stir until combined. Pour over the top of the berries in the slow cooker.

3. Cover and cook for 5 hours on low or 2½ hours on high. Remove the lid and skim off the excess butter. Replace the lid and continue cooking for another 30 minutes on high.

4. Allow to cool in the slow cooker and then gently remove the clafoutis by lifting up the sides of the baking paper. Serve with a drizzle of cream.

SWEET POTATO BROWNIES

Renee, our social media guru, took one of her favourite brownie recipes and made it work in the slow cooker. Yum!

SERVES 12–16

PREPARATION TIME
45 minutes

COOKING TIME
2½ hours on low
1½ hours on high

oil or butter, for greasing

3 tablespoons coconut flour

2 tablespoons raw cacao powder

½ teaspoon vanilla powder

¼ teaspoon gluten-free baking powder

¼ teaspoon ground cinnamon

pinch of salt

1 scoop (30 g) vanilla protein powder (optional)

50 g dark (85% cocoa) chocolate, chopped

1 cup (250 ml) unseasoned Sweet Potato Mash (see page 132) or 1 large sweet potato, baked until soft, skin removed

3 eggs, whisked

4 tablespoons melted coconut oil

⅓ cup (75 ml) rice malt syrup

1. Grease the slow-cooker insert and line with baking paper so that it reaches halfway up the sides.

2. In a bowl, combine the dry ingredients. In a separate bowl, whisk together all of the wet ingredients, including the sweet potato flesh, until combined.

3. Stir the dry ingredients into the wet and mix well. Pour into the prepared slow cooker and spread evenly.

4. Cover and cook for 2 hours on low or 1 hour on high. Remove the lid and cook for a further 30 minutes on low or until a skewer comes out clean when inserted. Gently remove the brownies by lifting up the sides of the baking paper. Set aside and allow to cool before serving.

PUMPKIN AND COURGETTE BREKKIE PUD

Our newest team member, Kate, came up with this deceptively healthy treat. It started out life as a breakfast loaf... but was happier as a 'pudding'. It's super yummy when topped with a dollop of natural yoghurt for breakfast or dessert.

SERVES 6–8

PREPARATION TIME
10 minutes

COOKING TIME
4 hours on low
2 hours on high

oil or butter, for greasing

2 cups (200 g) ground almonds

½ cup (60 g) gluten-free flour
(or regular if you prefer)

1 teaspoon baking powder

1 teaspoon sea salt

2 teaspoons ground cinnamon

¼ teaspoon ground nutmeg

125 g unsalted butter, softened

⅓ cup (75 ml) rice malt syrup

2 eggs

1 cup (250 ml) Pumpkin Purée
(see page 32)

1 cup (150 g) grated courgettes, drained

4 tablespoons unsweetened almond milk

1 teaspoon vanilla powder

½ cup (60 g) toasted pecans, roughly chopped

1. Grease the inside of the slow-cooker insert and line with baking paper so that it reaches about three-quarters of the way up the sides.

2. In a large bowl, combine the ground almonds, flour, baking powder, salt, cinnamon and nutmeg. Stir well and set aside.

3. In a separate bowl, beat the butter and rice malt syrup together with an electric beater. Add the eggs, one at a time, beating after each addition.

4. On low speed, beat in the pumpkin purée and courgettes, followed by the almond milk and vanilla. Slowly add the flour mixture and beat until the batter is just coming together.

5. Pour the batter into the prepared slow-cooker insert. Sprinkle the toasted pecans over the top. Cover and cook for 4 hours on low or 2 hours on high. Check the pudding by inserting a skewer into the centre – it should come out clean. If not, continue cooking on high with the lid off. Gently remove the brekkie pud by lifting up the sides of the baking paper. Set aside and allow to cool before serving.

> **TRICKY TIP**
>
> You could use sweet potato purée instead of pumpkin purée if you prefer.

INDEX

THANK YOU

Thanks to Stephanie Hinton and the I Quit Sugar team for recipe development. Thanks to the Pan Macmillan team and the fantastic food photography and styling that was carried out by Rob Palmer and Bernie Smithies.

Thank you to Matt Preston, Margaret Fulton and Kate Gibbs for allowing us to reproduce your delicious recipes here.

First published 2016 by Pan Macmillan Australia Pty Ltd

First published in the UK 2017 by Bluebird
an imprint of Pan Macmillan
20 New Wharf Road, London N1 9RR
Associated companies throughout the world
www.panmacmillan.com

ISBN 978-1-5098-4372-5

A CIP catalogue record for this book is available from the British Library.

Design by Elissa Webb, adapted from design by Lisa Valuyskaya
Printed and bound in China by 1010

Food styling and props by Bernadette Smithies
Food preparation by Sarah Mayoh

Visit **www.panmacmillan.com** to read more about all our books and to buy them. You will also find features, author interviews and news of any author events, and you can sign up for e-newsletters so that you're always first to hear about our new releases.